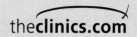

RADIOLOGIC
CLINICS
OF NORTH AMERICA

Update on Ultrasound

November 2006 • Volume 44 • Number 6

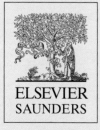

ELSEVIER
SAUNDERS

An imprint of Elsevier, Inc
PHILADELPHIA LONDON TORONTO MONTREAL SYDNEY TOKYO

W.B. SAUNDERS COMPANY
A Division of Elsevier Inc.

1600 John F. Kennedy Boulevard • Suite 1800 • Philadelphia, Pennsylvania 19103-2899

http://www.theclinics.com

RADIOLOGIC CLINICS OF NORTH AMERICA Volume 44, Number 6
November 2006 ISSN 0033-8389, ISBN 1-4160-4787-5; 978-1-4160-4787-2

Editor: Barton Dudlick

Reprints: For copies of 100 or more, of articles in this publication, please contact the Commercial Reprints Department, Elsevier Inc., 360 Park Avenue South, New York, New York 10010-1710. Tel.: (+1) 212-633-3813; Fax: (+1) 212-462-1935; E-mail: reprints@elsevier.com.

The ideas and opinions expressed in *Radiologic Clinics of North America* do not necessarily reflect those of the Publisher does not assume any responsibility for any injury and/or damage to persons or property arising out of or related to any use of the material contained in this periodical. The reader is advised to check the appropriate medical literature and the product information currently provided by the manufacturer of each drug to be administered to verify the dosage, the method and duration of administration, or contraindications, It is the responsibility of the treating physician or other health care professional, relying on independent experience and knowledge of the patient, to determine drug dosages and the best treatment for the patient. Mention of any product in this issue should not be construed as endorsement by the contributiors, editors, or the Publisher of the productor manufacturers' claims.

Radiologic Clinics of North America (ISSN 0033-8389) is published bimonthly in January, March, May, July, September, and November by Elsevier Inc., 360 Park Avenue South, New York, NY 10010-1710. Business and editorial offices: 1600 John F. Kenedy Boulevard, Suite 1800, Philadelphia, Pennsylvania 19103-2899. Customer Service Office: 6277 Sea Harbor Drive, Orlando, FL 32887-4800. Periodicals postage paid at New York, NY, and additional mailing offices. Subscription prices are USD 259 per year for US individuals, USD 385 per year for US institutions, USD 127 per year for US students and residents, USD 303 per year for Canadian individuals, USD 473 per year of Canadian institutions, USD 352 per year for international individuals, USD 473 per year for international institutions, and USD 171 per year for Canadian and foreign students/residents. To receive student and resident rate, orders must be accompanied by name of affiliated institution, date of term, and the signature of program/residency coordinatior on institution letterhead. Orders will be billed at individual rate until proof of status is received. Foreign air speed delivery is included in all Clinics subscriptionprices. All prices are subject to change without notice. **POSTMASTER:** Send address changes to *Radiologic Clinics of North America*, Elsevier Periodicals Customer Service, 6277 Sea Harbor Drive, Orlando, FL 32887-4800. **Customer Service: 1-800-654-2452 (US). From outside of the US, call (+1) 407-345-4000.**

Radiologic Clinics of North America also published in Greek Paschalidis Medical Publications, Athens, Greece.

Radiologic Clinics of North America is covered in *Index Medicus, EMBASE/Excerpta Medica, Current Contents/Life Sciences, Current Contents/Clinical Medicine, RSNA Index to Imaging Literature, BIOSIS, Science Citation Index,* and *ISI/BIOMED.*

Printed in the United States of America.

RADIOLOGIC CLINICS OF NORTH AMERICA NOVEMBER 2006

GOAL STATEMENT

The goal of the *Radiologic Clinics of North America* is to keep practicing radiologists and radiology residents up to date with current clinical practice in radiology by providing timely articles reviewing the state of the art in patient care.

ACCREDITATION

The *Radiologic Clinics of North America* is planned and implemented in accordance with the Essential Areas and Policies of the Accreditation Council for Continuing Medical Education (ACCME) through the joint sponsorship of the University of Virginia School of Medicine and Elsevier. The University of Virginia School of Medicine is accredited by the ACCME to provide continuing medical education for physicians.

The University of Virginia School of Medicine designates this educational activity for a maximum of 15 *AMA PRA Category 1 Credits*™. Physicians should only claim credit commensurate with the extent of their participation in the activity.

The American Medical Association has determined that physicians not licensed in the US who participate in this CME activity are eligible for 15 *AMA PRA Category 1 Credits*™.

Credit can be earned by reading the text material, taking the CME examination online at http://www.theclinics.com/home/cme, and completing the evaluation. After taking the test, you will be required to review any and all incorrect answers. Following completion of the test and evaluation, your credit will be awarded and you may print your certificate.

FACULTY DISCLOSURE/CONFLICT OF INTEREST

The University of Virginia School of Medicine, as an ACCME accredited provider, endorses and strives to comply with the Accreditation Council for Continuing Medical Education (ACCME) Standards of Commercial Support, Commonwealth of Virginia statutes, University of Virginia policies and procedures, and associated federal and private regulations and guidelines on the need for disclosure and monitoring of proprietary and financial interests that may affect the scientific integrity and balance of content delivered in continuing medical education activities under our auspices.

The University of Virginia School of Medicine requires that all CME activities accredited through this institution be developed independently and be scientifically rigorous, balanced and objective in the presentation/discussion of its content, theories and practices.

All authors/editors participating in an accredited CME activity are expected to disclose to the readers relevant financial relationships with commercial entities occurring within the past 12 months (such as grants or research support, employee, consultant, stock holder, member of speakers bureau, etc.). The University of Virginia School of Medicine will employ appropriate mechanisms to resolve potential conflicts of interest to maintain the standards of fair and balanced education to the reader. Questions about specific strategies can be directed to the Office of Continuing Medical Education, University of Virginia School of Medicine, Charlottesville, Virginia.

The authors/editors listed below have identified no financial or professional relationships for themselves or their spouse/partner:
Piyush K. Agarwal, MD; Shweta Bhatt, MD; Darren D. Brennan, MD; Jeanne Cullinan, MD; Vikram S. Dogra, MD; Barton Dudlick (Acquisitions Editor); Aimee D. Eyvazzadeh, MD; Suvranu Ganguli, MD; Jon Hyett, MD; Jo-Ann Johnson, MD, FRCSC; Robert A. Kane, MD, FACR; Jonathan B. Kruskal, MD, PhD; Deborah Levine, MD; Shannon Nedelka, MD; David A. Nyberg, MD; Raj Mohan Paspulati, MD; Maitray D. Patel, MD; Deborah J. Rubens, MD; Peter J. Strouse, MD; Srinivas Vourganti, MD; and, Therese M. Weber, MD.

The authors/editors listed below have identified the following financial or professional relationships for themselves or their spouse/partner:
Donald R. Bodner, MD is on the speakers bureau and has teaching engagements for Merck, Sanofi Aventis, Boeherger, Ingleheim, and Novartis; and, owns stock in Merck and Medtronics.
Steven R. Goldstein, MD is a consultant for Cook OB-GYN and Akrad Labs, a Cooper Company.
Vivienne Souter, MD has teaching engagements with Fetal Medicine Foundation/GeneCare.

Disclosure of Discussion of Non-FDA Approved Uses for Pharmaceutical and/or Medical Devices:
The University of Virginia School of Medicine, as an ACCME provider, requires that all authors identify and disclose any "off label" uses for pharmaceutical and medical device products. The University of Virginia School of Medicine recommends that each physician fully review all the available data on new products or procedures prior to clinical use.

TO ENROLL

To enroll in the *Radiologic Clinics of North America* Continuing Medical Education program, call customer service at **1-800-654-2452** or sign up online at http://www.theclinics.com/home/cme. The CME program is available to subscribers for an additional annual fee of $205.00.

UPDATE ON ULTRASOUND

CONTRIBUTORS

PIYUSH K. AGARWAL, MD
University Hospitals of Cleveland; Department of Urology, Case Western Reserve School of Medicine, Cleveland, Ohio

SHWETA BHATT, MD
Fellow, Department of Imaging Sciences, University of Rochester School of Medicine and Dentistry; Instructor, Department of Radiology, University of Rochester Medical Center, Rochester, New York

DONALD R. BODNER, MD
Professor of Urology, University Hospitals of Cleveland; Cleveland Department of Veterans, Affairs Medical Center; Department of Urology, Case Western Reserve School of Medicine, Cleveland, Ohio

DARREN D. BRENNAN, MD
Clinical Fellow of Radiology, Harvard Medical School; Department of Radiology, Beth Israel Deaconess Medical Center, Boston, Massachusetts

JEANNE CULLINAN, MD
Associate Professor, Department of Radiology, University of Rochester Medical Center, Rochester, New York

VIKRAM S. DOGRA, MD
Professor of Radiology and Associate Chair of Education and Research; Department of Imaging Sciences; Director, Division of Ultrasound, Department of Radiology, University of Rochester School of Medicine and Dentistry, Rochester, New York

AIMEE D. EYVAZZADEH, MD
Department of Obstetrics and Gynecology, Beth Israel Deaconess Medical Center, Boston, Massachusetts

STEVEN R. GOLDSTEIN, MD
Professor of Obstetrics and Gynecology; Director, Gynecologic Ultrasound; Co-Director, Bone Densitometry, New York University School of Medicine, New York, New York

SUVRANU GANGULI, MD
Clinical Fellow of Radiology, Harvard Medical School; Department of Radiology, Beth Israel Deaconess Medical Center, Boston, Massachusetts

JON HYETT, MD
Staff Specialist in Maternal and Fetal Medicine, Maternity Services, Royal Brisbane Women's Hospital, Herston, Australia

JO-ANN JOHNSON, MD, FRCSC
Professor of Obstetrics and Gynecology, Division of Maternal Fetal Medicine, Calgary, Alberta, Canada

ROBERT A. KANE, MD, FACR
Professor of Radiology, Harvard Medical School; and Co-Chief of Ultrasound, Department of Radiology, Beth Israel Deaconess Medical Center, Boston, Massachusetts

JONATHAN B. KRUSKAL, MD, PhD
Associate Professor of Radiology, Harvard Medical School; Chief, Abdominal Imaging, Department of Radiology, Beth Israel Deaconess Medical Center, Boston, Massachusetts

DEBORAH LEVINE, MD
Associate Professor, Department of Radiology, Harvard Medical School; Associate Radiologist and Chief of Academic Affairs, Beth Israel Deaconess Medical Center, Boston, Massachusetts

SHANNON NEDELKA, MD
Adjunct Assistant Professor, Department of Radiology, University of Rochester Medical Center, Rochester, New York

DAVID A. NYBERG, MD
Director, Fetal and Women's Center of Arizona, Scottsdale, Arizona

RAJ MOHAN PASPULATI, MD
Assistant Professor, Department of Radiology, University Hospitals of Cleveland, Case Western Reserve University, Cleveland, Ohio

MAITRAY D. PATEL, MD
Associate Professor of Radiology Mayo Clinic, Scottsdale, Arizona

DEBORAH J. RUBENS, MD
Department of Imaging Sciences, University of Rochester Medical Center, Rochester, New York

VIVIENNE SOUTER, MD
Good Samaritan Medical Center, Phoenix, Arizona

PETER J. STROUSE, MD
Associate Professor, Section of Pediatric Radiology, C.S. Mott Children's Hospital, Department of

Radiology, University of Michigan Health System, Ann Arbor, Michigan

SRINIVAS VOURGANTI, MD
University Hospitals of Cleveland; Professor, Department of Urology, Case Western Reserve School of Medicine, Cleveland, Ohio

THERESE M. WEBER, MD
Associate Professor, Department of Radiology, Wake Forest University School of Medicine, Winston-Salem, North Carolina

UPDATE ON ULTRASOUND

Volume 44 • Number 6 • November 2006

Contents

a Doppler signal, whether vascular, motion, or artifact. Color or power Doppler artifacts can be verified by their atypical spectral waveform. Some artifacts, such as aliasing (for rapid detection of stenoses or arteriovenous fistulae) and the twinkle artifact (for identification of renal calculi and verification of other stones or crystals), are extremely useful diagnostically. Careful attention to the technical parameters of frequency, gain, filter, and scale is required to correctly identify vascular patency or thrombosis, especially in slow flowing vessels.

First-Trimester Screening 837

David A. Nyberg, Jon Hyett, Jo-Ann Johnson, and Vivienne Souter

Screening for fetal chromosome abnormalities, particularly for trisomy 21, has made dramatic advances. Better screening demonstrates that "high-risk" patients—particularly over age 35—can have lower risk of defects than younger unscreened women. This has caused reduction of amniocentesis for older patients and made screening available for younger patients who have the universal 2% to 3% risk. This means lower procedural-related losses of normal fetuses, and better resource allocation. The trend toward first-trimester detection of structural defects continues; a normal survey is reassuring and helps exclude major defects. Based on screening results, patients can be triaged into early follow-up and possible amniocentesis at 14 to 16 weeks, or a later detailed anatomic survey at 18 to 20 weeks.

Imaging of Pelvic Pain in the First Trimester of Pregnancy 863

Aimee D. Eyvazzadeh and Deborah Levine

Pelvic pain during the first trimester of pregnancy can pose a challenge to the clinician. The noninvasive nature, safety, and reliability of ultrasonography make it the diagnostic method of choice for pregnant patients who have pelvic pain. Sonography provides information that allows for diagnosis of both pregnancy-related pain, such as a ruptured ectopic pregnancy, miscarriage, or threatened abortion; and may be useful in the diagnosis of pain unrelated to pregnancy, such as that seen in appendicitis and nephrolithiasis.

Practical Approach to the Adnexal Mass 879

Maitray D. Patel

Gynecologic sonography has matured into a highly effective and accurate tool enabling confident diagnosis of a variety of adnexal masses. Using a practical evidence-based approach, sonologists are well equipped to differentiate expected findings in the normal ovary from pathologic entities and can often generate specific conclusions regarding the cause of an adnexal mass. Mastery of the diagnostic strategies to use when an adnexal mass is identified and the sonographic patterns of various types of adnexal pathology contributes greatly to the proper and cost-effective care of a woman with an adnexal mass.

Abnormal Uterine Bleeding: The Role of Ultrasound 901

Steven R. Goldstein

Abnormal uterine bleeding is an important clinical concern and accounts for much medical intervention. This article presents an ultrasound-based approach to help exclude endometrial carcinoma and identify the source of bleeding for better clinical management. Saline infusion sonohysterography can help to triage patients to (1) no anatomic pathology, (2) globally thickened anatomic pathology that may be evaluated with blind endometrial sampling, or (3) focal abnormalities that must be evaluated under direct vision.

Sonographic Evaluation of the Child with Lower Abdominal or Pelvic Pain   911

Peter J. Strouse

At many centers, CT has become the primary imaging modality for children who have abdominal pain. CT, however, delivers a substantial radiation dose, which is of particular concern in the pediatric patient. In contrast, sonography does not expose the patient to ionizing radiation. Properly performed, sonography is capable of providing useful diagnostic information in the child who has lower abdominal or pelvic pain. In many children and with many disorders, sonography proves to be the only imaging modality that may be required. In this article, the usefulness of sonography in evaluating disorders producing lower abdominal or pelvic pain in a child is reviewed.

Intraoperative Laparoscopic Ultrasound   925

Suvranu Ganguli, Jonathan B. Kruskal, Darren D. Brennan, and Robert A. Kane

In parallel with the increasing move from open surgical procedures to laparoscopic approaches, laparoscopic ultrasound (LUS) is being used with increasing frequency to image normal structures and intra-abdominal pathology. Special transducers and scanning techniques are required to perform LUS with a different set of considerations. Within the spectrum of LUS applications, LUS is used to complement laparoscopy for oncology staging, to facilitate an array of surgical procedures, and to guide laparoscopic biopsies.

Index   937

ELSEVIER
SAUNDERS

RADIOLOGIC
CLINICS
OF NORTH AMERICA

Radiol Clin N Am 44 (2006) 763–775

Ultrasonographic Evaluation of Renal Infections

Srinivas Vourganti, MD[a], Piyush K. Agarwal, MD[a],
Donald R. Bodner, MD[a],*, Vikram S. Dogra, MD[b]

Medical ultrasonography dates back to the 1930s when it was adapted from technology used to test the strength of metal hulls of ships and applied to detect brain tumors [1]. Now with ultrasound being performed outside of the radiology suite and in emergency departments, patient clinics, hospital rooms, and doctors' offices, it compromises approximately 25% of all imaging studies performed worldwide [2]. Ultrasonography is noninvasive, rapid, readily available, portable, and offers no exposure to contrast or radiation. Furthermore, it is easily interpretable by physicians of several different disciplines and can result in quick diagnosis and treatment of potentially life-threatening conditions. Some of these conditions include severe kidney infections. This article focuses on reviewing ultrasound characteristics of various renal infections.

Ultrasound principles

Electric waveforms are applied to piezoelectric elements in the transducer causing them to vibrate

This article was originally published in *Ultrasound Clinics* 1:1, January 2006.
[a] Department of Urology, Case Western Reserve University School of Medicine and University Hospitals of Cleveland, 11100 Euclid Avenue, Cleveland, OH 44022, USA
[b] Department of Imaging Sciences, University of Rochester School of Medicine, 601 Elmwood Avenue, Box 648, Rochester, NY 14642, USA
* Corresponding author.
E-mail address: Dbodner180@aol.com (D.R. Bodner).

doi:10.1016/j.rcl.2006.10.001

and emit sound waves. The frequency range of the sound waves emitted is above the audible human range of 20 to 20,000 Hz (cycles per second). The sound waves generated range in frequency from 1 to 15 MHz (1,000,000 cycles per second) and are directed by the transducer into the body where they are either reflected, absorbed, or refracted based on the density of the different tissues the waves pass through. Sound passes through soft tissue at an average velocity of 1540 m/s. As the sound passes through tissues of differing densities, a portion of the sound waves is reflected back to the transducer and converted into electrical signals that are then amplified to produce an image. The strength of the returning sound waves or echoes is proportional to the difference in density between the two tissues forming the interface through which the sound waves are traveling [3]. If the sound waves encounter a homogenous fluid medium, such as the fluid in a renal cyst, they are transmitted through without interruption. As a result, no echoes are reflected back to the transducer, which produces an anechoic image [4]. Sound waves that are strongly reflected generate strong echoes and are visualized as bright white lines, creating a hyperechoic image.

In imaging the kidney, the highest frequency that produces adequate tissue penetration with a good resolution is selected. Tissue penetration is inversely related to the frequency of the transducer. Therefore, as the frequency increases, the depth of tissue penetration decreases. Conversely, image resolution is directly related to the frequency of the transducer. Therefore, as the frequency increases, the spatial resolution of the image increases [5]. To balance these two competing factors, a 3.5- or 5-MHz transducer is used to image the kidneys.

Ultrasound technique

Patients are imaged in the supine position and a coupling medium (eg, gel) is applied to the transducer to reduce the interference that may be introduced by air between the transducer and the skin. Generally a 3.5-MHz transducer is used, but a 5-MHz transducer can provide high-quality images in children or thin, adult patients. A breath-hold may be elicited by instructing the patient to hold their breath at maximal inspiration. This action will displace the kidneys inferiorly by approximately 2.5 cm and may provide a better view. The right kidney can be found by placing the transducer along the right lateral subcostal margin in the anterior axillary line during an inspiratory breath-hold. If the kidney cannot be imaged because of overlying bowel gas, then the probe can be moved laterally to the midaxillary line or the posterior axillary line.

Imaging the left kidney is often more challenging as it is located more superiorly, lacks an acoustic window such as the liver, and is covered by overlying gas from the stomach and small bowel. The left kidney can be localized by positioning the patient in the right lateral decubitus position and by placing the probe in the left posterior axillary line or in the left costovertebral angle [6]. The renal examination should include long-axis and transverse views of the upper poles, midportions, and lower poles. The cortex and renal pelvic regions should then be assessed. A maximum measurement of renal length should be recorded for both kidneys. Decubitus, prone, or upright positioning may provide better images of the kidney. When possible, renal echogenicity should be compared with the adjacent liver and spleen. The kidneys and perirenal regions should be assessed for abnormalities. Doppler may be used to differentiate vascular from nonvascular structures [7].

The normal kidney appears elliptical in longitudinal view [Fig. 1]. The right kidney varies in length from 8 to 14 cm, whereas the left kidney measures 7 to 12.5 cm. The kidneys are generally within 2 cm of each other in length and are 4 to 5 cm in width [8]. The renal cortex is homogenous and hypoechoic to the liver or spleen. The renal sinus contains the peripelvic fat; lymphatic and renal vessels; and the collecting system, and appears as a dense, central echogenic complex. The medulla can sometimes be differentiated from the cortex by the presence of small and round hypoechoic structures adjacent to the renal sinus [9].

Renal infections

Acute pyelonephritis

A patient who has acute pyelonephritis will classically appear with localized complaints of flank pain and costovertebral angle tenderness accompanied by generalized symptoms of fever, chills, nausea, and vomiting. In addition, these findings may be accompanied by further lower urinary tract symptoms, including dysuria, increased urinary frequency, and voiding urgency [10]. Laboratory abnormalities indicative of the underlying infection can be expected, including neutrophilic leukocytosis on the complete blood count and elevated erythrocyte sedimentation rate and serum C-reactive protein levels. If the infection is severe, it may interfere with renal function and cause an elevation of serum creatinine [11].

Evaluation of the urine will usually demonstrate frank pyuria with urinalysis demonstrating the presence of leukocyte esterase and nitrites and microscopic findings of numerous leukocytes and bacteria [12]. However, sterile urine can be seen

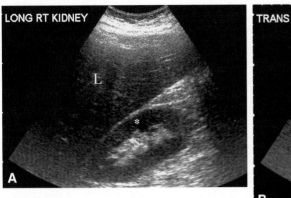
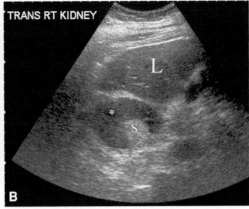

Fig. 1. Normal kidney. Longitudinal (*A*) and transverse (*B*) gray-scale sonogram of the right kidney demonstrates a hypoechoic renal cortex (*asterisk*) as compared with the liver, and a central hyperechoic renal sinus. L, liver; S, renal sinus.

despite acute pyelonephritis, especially in the setting of obstruction of the infected kidney [11]. Urine cultures, which should be collected before starting antibiotic therapy, will almost exclusively demonstrate ascending infection from gram-negative bacteria. Eighty percent of infections are caused by *Escherichia coli*. The remainder of cases is mostly caused by other gram-negative organisms, including *Klebsiella, Proteus, Enterobacter, Pseudomonas, Serratia,* and *Citrobacter*. With the exception of *Enterococcus faecalis* and *Staphylococcus epidermidis,* gram-positive bacteria are rarely the cause of acute pyelonephritis [10].

In addition to bacterial nephritis, fungal infections of the kidney are also possible. Infections with fungi are more commonly present in the setting of diabetes, immunosuppression, urinary obstruction, or indwelling urinary catheters [12]. Most commonly, *Candida* sp such as *Candida albicans* and *Candida tropicalis* are the causative organisms. In addition to the Candida, other fungi such as *Torulopsis glabrata, Aspergillus* sp, *Cryptococcus neoformans,* Zygomycetes (ie, *Rhizopus, Rhizomucor, Mucor,* and *Absidia* sp), and *Histoplasma capsulatum* may cause renal infections with less frequency. Clinically, these infections present similarly to bacterial infections. Diagnosis can be accomplished by evaluation of the urine where fungus can be found microscopically or through fungal cultures. These infections can cause the formation of fungal balls, otherwise called bezoars, in the renal pelvis and collecting system, which can contribute to obstruction [13].

Ultrasonographic features of acute pyelonephritis

Imaging is generally not necessary for the diagnosis and treatment of acute pyelonephritis. In uncomplicated cases, ultrasound imaging will usually find

a normal-appearing kidney [6]. However, in 20% of cases, generalized renal edema attributed to inflammation and congestion is present, which can be detected by ultrasound evaluation. This edema is formally defined as an overall kidney length in excess of 15 cm or, alternatively, an affected kidney that is at least 1.5 cm longer than the unaffected side [11]. Dilatation of the collecting system in the absence of appreciable obstructive cause may also be detected by ultrasound. A proposed mechanism of this dilatation is that bacterial endotoxins may inhibit normal ureteric peristaltic motion, resulting in hydroureter and hydronephrosis [10]. Parallel lucent streaks in the renal pelvis and ureter, which are most likely caused by mucosal edema, may also be detected on ultrasound. This finding is the equivalent of a striated nephrogram appearance on CT. Additionally, the renal parenchyma may be hypoechoic or attenuated. In cases of fungal infection, collections of air may be seen in the bladder or collecting system as the fungus may be gas-forming. In addition, ultrasonography may demonstrate evidence of fungal debris in the collecting system, such as a bezoar and consequent obstruction [Fig. 2] [13].

In relation to other modalities of renal imaging (Tc-99m dimercaptosuccinic acid [DMSA] scintigraphy, spiral CT, and MR), ultrasound has been found to be less sensitive and specific in the diagnosis of acute pyelonephritis [14]. In the pediatric population, where a missed diagnosis can mean irreversible damage, Tc-99m DMSA scintigraphy is still considered the gold standard of imaging [15]. Improvements in ultrasound techniques by way of power Doppler ultrasonography have resulted in better imaging than B-mode ultrasonography alone, but do not improve on the accuracy of Tc-99m DMSA scintigraphy [16]. Some authors suggest that although power Doppler cannot replace

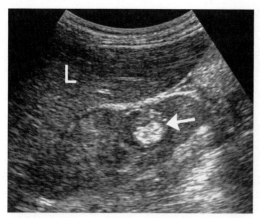

Fig. 2. Fungal ball. Longitudinal gray-scale sonogram of the right kidney in an immunocompromised patient demonstrates an echogenic mass (*arrow*) within a dilated calyx confirmed to be a fungus ball. L, liver.

Tc-99m DMSA scintigraphy because of its lack of sensitivity, a positive power Doppler ultrasound finding can obviate the need for further imaging [17]. In addition, when combined with concomitant laboratory findings such as an elevated serum C-reactive protein level, sensitivity and specificity can be improved, and results correlate with those of DMSA findings [18]. However, suggestions that ultrasound can serve as a replacement to other more sensitive modalities in the detection of acute pyelonephritis remain controversial.

Acute focal and multifocal pyelonephritis (acute lobar nephronia)

Acute focal and multifocal pyelonephritis occur when infection is confined to a single lobe or occurs in multiple lobes, respectively, of the kidney. More common in patients who have diabetes and those who are immunosuppressed, these infections will present with clinical features similar to acute pyelonephritis. However, the patient will generally experience more severe symptoms than patients who have uncomplicated pyelonephritis. In addition,

focal pyelonephritis commonly progresses to sepsis [10]. Treatment is similar to other complicated cases of acute pyelonephritis, with 7 days of parenteral antibiotics followed by a 7-day course of oral antibiotics [11].

Ultrasonographic features of acute focal and multifocal pyelonephritis

In imaging acute focal pyelonephritis, it is important to differentiate it from the more severe case of a renal abscess that requires more aggressive management. On ultrasound, the classic description of acute focal pyelonephritis is of a sonolucent mass that is poorly marginated with occasional low-amplitude echoes that disrupt the corticomedullary junction [Fig. 3] [6]. The absence of a distinct wall is a defining feature that differentiates focal nephritis from the more serious renal abscess [19]. Farmer and colleagues suggest that an ultrasonographic appearance of increased echogenicity, rather than sonolucent masses, may also be commonly seen in focal nephritis [20]. The ultrasound evaluation should be complemented with a CT evaluation, which is more sensitive in detecting focal pyelonephritis [21]. CT findings demonstrate a lobar distribution of inflammation that appears as a wedge-shaped area of decreased contrast enhancement on delayed images. In more severe disease, a hypodense mass lesion can be seen [19]. The radiologic appearance of multifocal disease is identical to focal disease except that it is seen in more than one lobe.

Renal abscess

Before the advent of antibiotics, most abscesses in the kidney were caused by hematogenous spread (usually of *Staphylococcus* sp) from distant sites. These renal carbuncles would be associated with a history (often remote) of a gram-positive infection elsewhere in the body, such as a carbuncle of the skin [10]. With antibiotic therapy now common, renal carbuncles are now rare, and instances

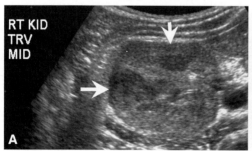

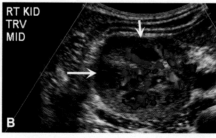

Fig. 3. Pyelonephritis. Transverse gray-scale (*A*) and color flow Doppler (*B*) sonography of the right kidney demonstrate two wedge-shaped areas of decreased echogenicity (*arrows*) in the renal cortex with absence of color flow, consistent with multifocal pyelonephritis.

of renal abscess are now primarily caused by ascending infection with enteric, aerobic, gram-negative bacilli, including *Escherichia coli*, *Klebsiella* sp, and *Proteus* sp [19]. Patients are at an increased risk for these abscesses if they have a complicated urinary tract infection (with stasis or obstruction), are diabetic, or are pregnant [10]. Patients will present with fever, chills, and pain in their back and abdomen. In addition, many will have symptoms characteristic of a urinary tract infection, such as dysuria, frequency, urgency, and suprapubic pain. Constitutional symptoms of malaise and weight loss may also be seen [10]. Laboratory studies will demonstrate a leukocytosis. In nearly all renal carbuncles, and up to 30% of gram-negative abscesses, the abscess does not involve the collecting system and urine cultures will be negative [19]. In general, any positive urine culture will match the blood culture in the setting of an ascending gram-negative abscess. In the event of a gram-positive renal carbuncle, the urine culture and blood cultures may isolate different organisms from one another [10].

The management of renal abscesses is generally dictated by their size. Small abscesses (smaller than 3 cm) are treated conservatively with observation and parenteral antibiotics. Similar-sized lesions in patients who are immunocompromised may be treated more aggressively with some form of abscess drainage. Lesions between 3 and 5 cm are often treated with percutaneous drainage. Any abscess larger than 5 cm usually requires surgical drainage.

Ultrasonographic features of renal abscess

Ultrasound is particularly useful in the diagnosis of renal abscess [19]. It usually shows an enlarged kidney with distortion of the normal renal contour [Fig. 4]. Acutely, the abscess will appear to have indistinct margins with edema in the surrounding renal parenchyma. However, after convalescence, it will appear as a fluid-filled mass with a distinct wall. This clear margin helps to distinguish this entity from the less severe focal nephritis. Once identified by ultrasound, CT scanning with contrast enhancement can better characterize these lesions. The abscess will be seen as a round or oval

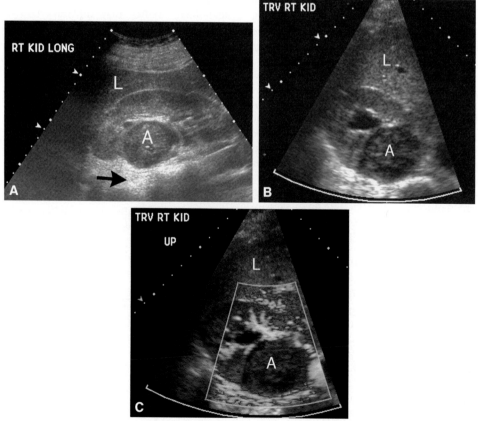

Fig. 4. Renal abscess. Longitudinal (*A*) and transverse (*B*) gray-scale ultrasound of the right kidney reveal presence of a well-defined hypoechoic lesion (*A*) near the superior pole, with posterior through transmission (*arrow*). Corresponding power Doppler image (*C*) demonstrates an increased peripheral vascularity. L, Liver.

parenchymal mass with decreased levels of attenuation. A ring circumscribing the lesion will form with contrast enhancement ("ring sign") because of the increased vascularity of the abscess wall [10]. In many instances, it will be difficult to definitively distinguish a renal abscess from a renal tumor. In these cases, radiologic-guided drainage with analysis of fluid can be helpful in establishing the diagnosis.

Emphysematous pyelonephritis

Emphysematous pyelonephritis is a complication of acute pyelonephritis in which gas-forming organisms infect renal parenchyma. It is usually caused by *E coli* (70% of cases), but *Klebsiella pneumoniae* and *Proteus mirabilis* can cause emphysematous pyelonephritis with less frequency [22]. A necrotizing infection occurs in the renal parenchyma and perirenal tissues in which tissue is used as a substrate with carbon dioxide gas released as a byproduct. Clinically, this infection usually occurs in patients who have diabetes in the setting of urinary tract obstruction. Women are affected more than men. There have been no reported cases in children. Nearly all patients will present with the following triad of symptoms: fever, vomiting, and flank pain. Pneumaturia can be seen when the collecting system is involved. However, focal physical findings are commonly absent [11].

Once discovered, prompt treatment is imperative. Management should begin with supportive care, management of diabetes, and relief of any underlying obstruction. If infection is discovered in one kidney, the contralateral kidney should also be thoroughly investigated, as bilateral involvement is seen in up to 10% of cases. The classic management for emphysematous pyelonephritis is administration of broad-spectrum antibiotics along with emergent nephrectomy [10]. Despite this aggressive therapy, mortality is seen in 30% to 40% of cases.

Ultrasonographic findings of emphysematous pyelonephritis

Emphysematous pyelonephritis is diagnosed by demonstrating gas in the renal parenchyma with or without extension into the perirenal tissue [10]. Ultrasound examination will characteristically show an enlarged kidney containing high-amplitude echoes within the renal parenchyma, often with low-level posterior dirty acoustic shadowing known as reverberation artifacts [Fig. 5]. However, the depth of parenchymal involvement may be underestimated during the ultrasound examination. Consequently, multiple renal stones may also manifest as echogenic foci without "clean"

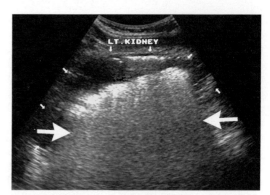

Fig. 5. Emphysematous pyelonephritis. Longitudinal gray-scale sonogram of the left kidney (*small arrows*) demonstrates air within the renal parenchyma with reverberation artifact (*large arrows*).

posterior shadowing [23,24]. The isolated presence of gas within the collecting system can be seen after many interventional procedures and should not be confused with emphysematous pyelonephritis. In these cases, an evaluation using CT is always warranted and is considered the ideal study to visualize the extent and amount of gas. In addition, CT can identify any local destruction to perirenal tissues. Radiologic studies play an important role in evaluation of the effectiveness of therapy in emphysematous pyelonephritis. As carbon dioxide is rapidly absorbed, any persistence of gas after 10 days of appropriate treatment is indicative of failed therapy [10].

Pyonephrosis

Pyonephrosis is a suppurative infection in the setting of hydronephrosis, which occurs as the result of obstruction. The renal pelvis and calyces become distended with pus [6]. Patients present with fevers, chills, and flank pain. Because of the obstruction, bacteriuria can be absent. It is imperative that this obstruction is relieved through a nephrostomy or ureteral stent. If untreated, pyonephrosis can cause destruction of renal parenchyma and irreversible loss of renal function [10].

Ultrasonographic features of pyonephrosis

Ultrasound findings are useful in early and accurate diagnosis of pyonephrosis. On examination, persistent echoes are seen in a dilated collecting system [Fig. 6]. This echogenicity is caused by debris in the collecting system, and is therefore seen in dependent areas of the collecting system. Shifts in this debris can sometimes be appreciated if the patient is asked to change positions during the ultrasound examination. In addition, air can be seen in these infections. In this event, strong echoes

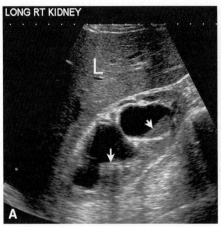
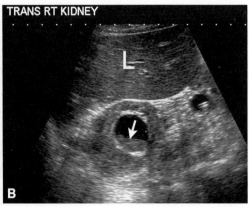

Fig. 6. Pyohydronephrosis. Longitudinal (*A*) and transverse (*B*) gray-scale sonogram of the right kidney demonstrate an enlarged hydronephrotic kidney with a fluid-fluid level (*arrows*) in the dilated calyces secondary to pus appearing as echogenic debris. L, liver.

with acoustic shadowing can be seen behind the affected area of the collecting system [11].

Xanthogranulomatous pyelonephritis

Xanthogranulomatous pyelonephritis (XGP) is a rare inflammatory condition that is seen in the setting of long-term and recurrent obstruction from nephrolithiasis accompanied by infection. It results in the irreversible destruction of renal parenchyma. This damage begins in the renal pelvis and calyces and eventually extends into the renal parenchyma and can occur in either a diffuse or segmental pattern [11]. Though the cause of XGP is unknown, it is thought that the inflammatory process that occurs in response to tissue damage by bacterial infection (usually *Proteus mirabilis* or *E coli*) results in the deposition of lipid-laden histiocytes at the site of infection. These macrophages, or xanthoma cells, along with other inflammatory cells result in the formation of fibrous tissue. This granulomatous process eventually replaces the adjacent normal renal parenchyma and adjacent renal tissue [10].

Clinically, XGP is seen more commonly in women than men. Incidence peaks during the fifth to sixth decade of life. Patients who have diabetes are predisposed to the formation of XGP. Symptoms include those that suggest underlying chronic infection in the setting of obstruction, such as fever, flank pain, persistent bacteriuria, or history of recurrent infected nephrolithiasis. XGP results in the irregular enlargement of the kidney and is often misdiagnosed as a tumor. Even by pathologic examination, XGP can closely resemble malignancy, such as renal cell carcinoma. Definitive diagnosis is often made only after surgical removal, which allows thorough pathologic examination. Treatment of XGP involves surgical removal of the entire

inflammatory process. Limited disease may be amenable to partial nephrectomy; however, more widespread XGP requires total nephrectomy and removal of the involved adjacent tissue [11]. Though classic management suggests that conservative intervention through simple incision and drainage commonly results in further complications, some investigators suggest this course in cases of limited focal disease [25].

Ultrasonographic features of xanthogranulomatous pyelonephritis

Definitive preoperative diagnosis is extremely difficult to establish in XGP. By ultrasound evaluation, multiple hypoechoic round masses can be seen in the affected kidney. These masses can demonstrate internal echoes and can be abscesses (with increased sound through-transmission) or solid granulomatous processes (with decreased sound through-transmission) [11]. Global enlargement with relative preservation of the renal contour can be seen with diffuse disease. However, in focal or segmental XGP a mass-like lesion may be appreciated. In addition, evidence of obstruction and renal calculus is commonly seen (85%) [26]. In general, CT evaluation is considered more informative than ultrasound in describing XGP. A large reniform mass within the renal pelvis tightly surrounding a central calcification is seen on CT imaging [10]. Dilated calyces and abscesses that replace normal renal parenchyma will appear as water-density masses. Calcifications and low attenuation areas attributed to lipid-rich xanthogranulomatous tissue may be seen within the masses [27]. If contrast is used, a blush is seen in the walls of these masses because of their vascularity. This enhancement, which is limited to the mass wall only, will help distinguish XGP from renal tumors and other inflammatory processes that do enhance throughout [11].

Renal malakoplakia

Renal malakoplakia is a rare inflammatory disorder associated with a chronic coliform gram-negative urinary tract infection (usually *E coli*) resulting in the deposition of soft, yellow-brown plaques within the bladder and upper urinary tract. The cause is thought to be abnormal macrophage function that causes incomplete intracellular bacterial lysis. This lysis results in the deposition of histiocytes, called von Hansemann cells, that are filled with these bacteria and bacterial fragments. The bacteria form a nidus for calcium phosphate crystals, which form small basophilic bodies called Michaelis-Gutmann bodies [10].

Clinically, malakoplakia of the urinary tract usually occurs in women. Most patients are older than 50 years. There is often an underlying condition compromising the immune system, such as diabetes, immunosuppression, or the presence of a chronic debilitating disease. Symptoms of a urinary tract infection may be present, such as fever, irritative voiding symptoms, and flank pain. In addition, a palpable mass may be appreciated [11]. If the disease involves the bladder, symptoms of bladder irritability and hematuria may be seen.

Ultrasonographic features of malakoplakia

Imaging findings of malakoplakia are nonspecific and can often mimic other pathology, such as renal tumors [28]. The most common ultrasonographic feature of renal malakoplakia is diffuse enlargement of the affected kidney [29]. Increased echogenicity of the renal parenchyma can be seen because of a confluence of the plaques [10]. In addition, hypoechoic lesions and distortion of parenchymal echoes may be appreciated [29].

Hydatid disease of the kidney (renal echinococcosis)

Echinococcosis is a parasitic infection that is most commonly seen in South Africa, the Mediterranean, Eastern Europe, Australia, and New Zealand. It is caused by the tapeworm *Echinococcus granulosis*. Although the adult form is zoonotic, mostly found in the intestines of dogs, humans may serve as an intermediate host of this parasite while it is in the larval stage [11]. Infection more commonly manifests in the liver and lungs, with only 4% of echinococcosis involving the kidney, because the larvae, which originally invade the body through the gastrointestinal tract, must first escape sequestration in the liver and subsequently the lungs. Only after these two defenses are surpassed are the larvae able to gain widespread access to the systemic circulation, and correspondingly, the kidneys [30].

The offending lesion will most commonly form as a solitary mass in the renal cortex. It is divided into three distinct zones. The outermost adventitial layer consists of host fibroblasts that may become calcified. A middle laminated layer consists of hyaline that surrounds a third inner germinal layer. The germinal layer is composed of nucleated epithelium and is where the echinococcal larvae reproduce. The larvae attach to the surrounding germinal layer and form brood capsules. These brood capsules grow in size and will remain connected to the germinal layer by a pedicle for nutrition. The core of this hydatid cyst contains detached brood capsules (daughter cysts), free larvae, and fluid, a combination known as hydatid sand [10].

Clinically, most patients who have renal echinococcosis are asymptomatic, especially in the beginning stages of the disease process because the cyst starts small and grows at a rate of only 1 cm annually. Because of their focal nature, small hydatid cysts will rarely affect renal function. As the lesion progresses, a mass effect will contribute to symptoms of dull flank pain, hematuria, and a palpable mass on examination [10]. If the cyst ruptures, a strong antigenic immune response ensues with possible urticaria and even anaphylaxis [30]. If a cyst ruptures into the collecting system, the patient will develop symptoms of hydatiduria, including renal colic and passage of urinary debris resembling grape skins [11].

Treatment of echinococcal disease in the kidney is primarily surgical. Medical therapy with antiparasitic agents, such as mebendazole, has been shown to be largely unsuccessful. In removing a cyst, great care must be taken to avoid its rupture. Any release of cyst contents can contribute to anaphylaxis. In addition, the release of the larvae can result in the dissemination of the disease. In the event of rupture, or if resection of the entire cyst is not possible, careful aspiration of the cyst is indicated. After the contents of the cyst are removed, an infusion of an antiparasitic agent (eg, 30% sodium chloride, 0.5% silver nitrate, 2% formalin, or 1% iodine) is reinfused into the cyst [11].

Ultrasonographic features of renal echinococcosis

Ultrasonographic findings of echinococcosis demonstrate different findings based on the age, extent, and complications of the hydatid cyst [30]. These lesions can be classified by the Gharbi ultrasonographic classification [Table 1] [30]. The Gharbi

Table 1: Gharbi ultrasonographic classification of hyatid cysts

Type	Pathology	Frequency	Ultrasonographic findings
I	Discrete univesicular mass	22%	Liquid-filled cyst with parietal echo backing
II	Univesicular mass with detached membranes	4%	Liquid-filled cyst with ultrasonographic water lily sign
III	Multivesicular mass	54%	Partitioned cyst with a spoke wheel appearance
IV	Heterogenous mass	12%	Heterogeneous echo structure with mixed solid and liquid components
V	Heterogenous mass with calcifications	8%	Dense reflections with a posterior shade cone caused by calcifications

classification assists in the characterization of renal masses that are caused by hydatid disease. Higher Gharbi type corresponds with further disease progression. Consequently, Gharbi type I cysts are most commonly seen in children. Accordingly, Gharbi types III through V are consistent with more advanced disease and are seen almost exclusively in adults. Most common are the Gharbi type III cysts, which are multivesicular masses that can be detected on ultrasound as a partitioned cyst with a spoke wheel appearance [Fig. 7A, B] [31]. Changes in patient position can cause any hydatid sand that is present to be disturbed and will result in the shifting of bright echoes within the mass. This finding has been described as the snowstorm sign [11,32]. Less commonly seen are the univesicular Gharbi type I and type II cysts, which demonstrate less disease progression and are seen more commonly in young adults and children. Type I cysts are well-limited liquid cysts that can

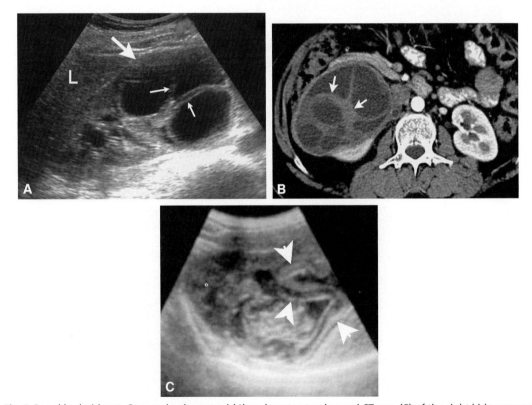

Fig. 7. Renal hydatid cyst. Gray-scale ultrasound (*A*) and contrast-enhanced CT scan (*B*) of the right kidney reveal a well-defined cystic lesion (*large arrow*) with multiple internal septae (*small arrows*) suggestive of a hydatid cyst with multiple daughter cysts. (Courtesy of SA Merchant, India.) (*C*) Gray-scale sonography of the right kidney on a different patient demonstrates the floating membranes (*arrowheads*) of the hydatid cyst following rupture of the cyst, referred to as the water lily sign. (Courtesy of Ercan Kocakoc, Turkey.)

be differentiated from simple nonhydatid cysts by the presence of a parietal echo. Gharbi type II cysts demonstrate a detached and floating membrane that is pathognomonic for hydatid disease. This detachment of the membranes inside the cyst has been referred to as the ultrasound water lily sign because of its resemblance to the radiographic water lily sign seen in pulmonary cysts [Fig. 7C] [33,34]. In contrast, the Gharbi type IV and V cysts demonstrate more advanced disease and are correspondingly seen in older patients. Gharbi type IV hydatid cysts will demonstrate heterogeneity of echo structure with a combination of liquid and solid cyst contents. Gharbi type V hydatid cysts are calcified and will show dense reflections with a posterior shade cone. The varying echogenic aspects of these type IV and V lesions make diagnosis by ultrasound more difficult [30]. In these cases, CT studies can aid in characterization. On CT, the presence of smaller round daughter cysts within the mother cysts can help differentiate hydatid lesions from other similar appearing pathology, such as simple cysts, abscesses, and necrotic neoplasm [10].

Renal tuberculosis

Tuberculosis is an infection caused by *Mycobacterium tuberculosis*. Typically acquired by inhalation, exposure initially results in a primary infection with a silent bacillemia. This infection will result in systemic dissemination of mycobacteria. Latent foci may result in kidney lesions many years following primary infection, though only 5% of patients who have active tuberculosis will have cavitary lesions in the urinary tract [11].

Clinically, this infection presents in younger patients, with 75% of those affected being younger than 50 years. Renal tuberculosis should be considered in any patient who has a diagnosed history of tuberculosis. Often patients will present asymptomatically, even in cases of advanced disease. If disease involves the bladder, symptoms of urinary frequency may result. One quarter of patients will

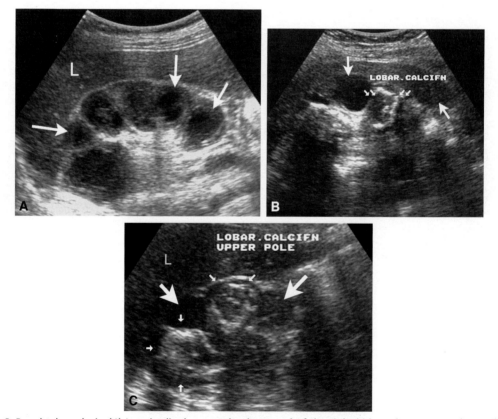

Fig. 8. Renal tuberculosis. (*A*) Longitudinal gray-scale ultrasound of the right kidney demonstrates hypoechoic areas (*arrows*) in the renal cortex suggestive of lobar caseation in this known case of tuberculosis. Longitudinal gray-scale sonography (*B, C*) of the kidney in another patient who has renal tuberculosis demonstrates hypoechoic areas of caseous necrosis (*large arrows*) with dense peripheral calcification (*small arrows*) with posterior acoustic shadowing. (Panels B, C, Courtesy of SA Merchant, Mumbai, India.)

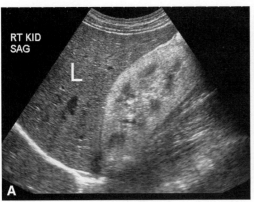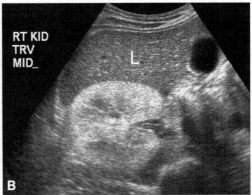

Fig. 9. HIV nephropathy. Longitudinal (*A*) and transverse (*B*) gray-scale sonograms of the right kidney in young man who has no known history of medical disease reveals an enlarged, markedly echogenic kidney (bilateral; left not shown) with loss of corticomedullary differentiation and obliteration of sinus fat suggestive of HIV-nephropathy. Subsequently confirmed by histopathology. L, liver.

present with findings of a unilateral poorly functioning kidney. Other suspicious findings include chronic cystitis or epididymitis that is recalcitrant to treatment; firm seminal vesicles on digital rectal examination; or a chronic fistula tract that forms at surgical sites. Diagnosis of urinary tract tuberculosis can be established through a urine culture that demonstrates growth of *M tuberculosis*.

Ultrasonographic features of renal tuberculosis

Early findings of urinary tract tuberculosis are best characterized by intravenous urography. Initially, cavities appear as small irregularities of the minor calyces. These irregular changes are classically described as "feathery" and "moth-eaten." As disease progresses, it extends from the calyces into the underlying renal parenchyma. Calcifications may be appreciated in these areas of caseating necrosis. In addition, tuberculosis involvement of the ureter can result in ureteral strictures, which cause a urographic appearance of a rigid, irregular, "pipe-stem" ureter [11]. Ultrasound findings in the diagnosis of renal tuberculosis have traditionally been described as limited. However, recent reports describe the role of high-resolution ultrasonography in characterizing late and chronic changes in renal tuberculosis [35]. Granulomatous mass lesions in the renal parenchyma can be seen as masses of mixed echogenicity, with or without necrotic areas of caseation and calcifications [Fig. 8]. Mucosal thickening and stenosis of the calyces is detectable by ultrasonography. In addition, findings of mucosal thickening of the renal pelvis and ureter, ureteral stricture, and hydronephrosis are seen. Finally, bladder changes such as mucosal thickening and reduced capacity are commonly detectable.

HIV-associated nephropathy

Renal disease is a common complication in patients who have HIV. This complication can result primarily from direct kidney infection with HIV or secondarily from adverse effects of the medications used to treat HIV. HIV-associated nephropathy (HIVAN) accounts for approximately 10% of new end stage renal disease cases in the United States. Patients who have HIVAN are not typically hypertensive.

Ultrasonographic features of HIV-associated nephropathy

Sonography is a critical component in the evaluation of HIVAN. The major sonographic findings include increased cortical echogenicity, decreased corticomedullary definition, and decreased renal sinus fat [Fig. 9]. Renal size may be enlarged [36,37]. The increased cortical echogenicity is attributable to prominent interstitial expansion by cellular infiltrate and markedly dilated tubules containing voluminous casts. Histologically, HIVAN demonstrates tubular epithelial cell damage, glomerulosclerosis, and tubulointerstitial scarring [38]. Most patients who have HIVAN have proteinuria secondary to tubular epithelial cell damage. In the presence of marked increased cortical echogenicity in a young patient who has known history of medical renal disease, HIVAN must be considered.

Summary

The growing ubiquity, well-established safety, and cost-effectiveness of ultrasound imaging have cemented its role in the diagnosis of renal infectious diseases. It is imperative that all practitioners of renal medicine understand the ultrasonographic manifestations of these diseases, as early diagnosis and treatment are the cornerstones of avoidance of long-term morbidity and mortality. If the strengths and limitations of ultrasonography are understood properly, a practitioner will be able to achieve the quickest and safest diagnosis with the minimal amount of further invasive imaging. The advent of new ultrasonographic techniques may allow it to serve a more central role in the diagnosis and characterization of renal infections.

References

[1] Newman PG, Rozycki GS. The history of ultrasound. Surg Clin North Am 1998;78(2):179–95.

[2] Harvey CJ, Pilcher JM, Eckersley RJ, et al. Advances in ultrasound. Clin Radiol 2002;57(3):157–77.

[3] McAchran SE, Dogra VS, Resnick MI. Office based ultrasound for urologists. Part I: ultrasound physics, and of the kidney and bladder. AUA Update 2004;23:226–31.

[4] Spirnak JP, Resnick MI. Ultrasound. In: Gillenwater JY, Grayhack JT, Howards SS, et al, editors. Adult & pediatric urology. 4th edition. Philadelphia: Lippincott, Williams & Williams; 2002. p. 165–93.

[5] Smith RS, Fry WR. Ultrasound instrumentation. Surg Clin North Am 2004;84(4):953–71.

[6] Noble VE, Brown DF. Renal ultrasound. Emerg Med Clin North Am 2004;22(3):641–59.

[7] Grant EG, Barr LL, Borgstede J, et al. AIUM standard for the performance of an ultrasound examination of the abdomen or retroperitoneum. American Institute of Ultrasound in Medicine. J Ultrasound Med 2002;21(10):1182–7.

[8] Brandt TD, Neiman HL, Dragowski MJ, et al. Ultrasound assessment of normal renal dimensions. J Ultrasound Med 1982;1(2):49–52.

[9] Horstman W, Watson L. Ultrasound of the genitourinary tract. In: Resnick MI, Older RA, editors. Diagnosis of genitourinary disease. 2nd edition. New York: Thieme; 1997. p. 79–130.

[10] Schaeffer AJ. Infections of the urinary tract. In: Walsh PC, Retik AB, Vaughn ED, et al, editors. Campbell's urology. 8th edition. Philadelphia: Elsevier; 2002. p. 516–602.

[11] Schaeffer AJ. Urinary tract infections. In: Gillenwater JY, Grayhack JT, Howards SS, et al, editors. Adult & pediatric urology. 4th edition. Philadelphia: Lippincott, Williams & Williams; 2002. p. 289–351.

[12] Ramakrishnan K, Scheid DC. Diagnosis and management of acute pyelonephritis in adults. Am Fam Physician 2005;71(5):933–42.

[13] Wise G. Fungal and actinomycotic infections of the genitourinary system. In: Walsh PC, Retik AB, Vaughn ED, et al, editors. Campbell's urology. 8th edition. Philadelphia: Elsevier; 2002. p. 797–827.

[14] Majd M, Nussbaum Blask AR, Markle BM, et al. Acute pyelonephritis: comparison of diagnosis with 99mTc-DMSA, SPECT, spiral CT, MR imaging, and power Doppler US in an experimental pig model. Radiology 2001;218(1):101–8.

[15] Johansen TE. The role of imaging in urinary tract infections. World J Urol 2004;22(5):392–8.

[16] Berro Y, Baratte B, Seryer D, et al. Comparison between scintigraphy, B-mode, and power Doppler sonography in acute pyelonephritis in children. J Radiol 2000;81(5):523–7.

[17] Bykov S, Chervinsky L, Smolkin V, et al. Power Doppler sonography versus Tc-99m DMSA scintigraphy for diagnosing acute pyelonephritis in children: are these two methods comparable? Clin Nucl Med 2003;28(3):198–203.

[18] Wang YT, Chiu NT, Chen MJ, et al. Correlation of renal ultrasonographic findings with inflammatory volume from dimercaptosuccinic acid renal scans in children with acute pyelonephritis. J Urol 2005;173(1):190–4.

[19] Dembry LM, Andriole VT. Renal and perirenal abscesses. Infect Dis Clin North Am 1997;11(3):663–80.

[20] Farmer KD, Gellett LR, Dubbins PA. The sonographic appearance of acute focal pyelonephritis 8 years experience. Clin Radiol 2002;57(6):483–7.

[21] Cheng CH, Tsau YK, Hsu SY, et al. Effective ultrasonographic predictor for the diagnosis of acute lobar nephronia. Pediatr Infect Dis J 2004;23(1):11–4.

[22] Stone SC, Mallon WK, Childs JM, et al. Emphysematous pyelonephritis: clues to rapid diagnosis in the Emergency Department. J Emerg Med 2005;28(3):315–9.

[23] Narlawar RS, Raut AA, Nagar A, et al. Imaging features and guided drainage in emphysematous pyelonephritis: a study of 11 cases. Clin Radiol 2004;59(2):192–7.

[24] Best CD, Terris MK, Tacker JR, et al. linical and radiological findings in patients with gas forming renal abscess treated conservatively. J Urol 1999;162(4):1273–6.

[25] Bingol-Kologlu M, Ciftci AO, Senocak ME, et al. Xanthogranulomatous pyelonephritis in children: diagnostic and therapeutic aspects. Eur J Pediatr Surg 2002;12(1):42–8.

[26] Tiu CM, Chou YH, Chiou HJ, et al. Sonographic features of xanthogranulomatous pyelonephritis. J Clin Ultrasound 2001;29(5):279–85.

[27] Kim JC. US and CT findings of xanthogranulomatous pyelonephritis. Clin Imaging 2001;25(2):118–21.

[28] Evans NL, French J, Rose MB. Renal malacoplakia: an important consideration in the differential diagnosis of renal masses in the presence of Escherichia coli infection. Br J Radiol 1998;71(850):1083–5.

[29] Venkatesh SK, Mehrotra N, Gujral RB. Sonographic findings in renal parenchymal malacoplakia. J Clin Ultrasound 2000;28(7):353–7.

[30] Zmerli S, Ayed M, Horchani A, et al. Hydatid cyst of the kidney: diagnosis and treatment. World J Surg 2001;25(1):68–74.

[31] von Sinner WN. New diagnostic signs in hydatid disease; radiography, ultrasound, CT and MRI correlated to pathology. Eur J Radiol 1991;12(2): 150–9.

[32] Marti-Bonmati L, Menor Serrano F. Complications of hepatic hydatid cysts: ultrasound, computed tomography, and magnetic resonance diagnosis. Gastrointest Radiol 1990;15(2):119–25.

[33] Beggs I. The radiology of hydatid disease. AJR Am J Roentgenol 1985;145(3):639–48.

[34] Moguillanski SJ, Gimenez CR, Villavicencio RL. Radiología de la hidatidosis abdominal. In: Stoopen ME, Kimura K, Ros PR, editors. Radiología e imagen diagnóstica y terapeútica: abdomen, Vol. 2. Philadelphia: Lippincott Williams & Wilkins; 1999. p. 47–72.

[35] Vijayaraghavan SB, Kandasamy SV, Arul M, et al. Spectrum of high-resolution sonographic features of urinary tuberculosis. J Ultrasound Med 2004;23(5):585–94.

[36] Di Fiori JL, Rodrigue D, Kaptein EM, et al. Diagnostic sonography of HIV-associated nephropathy: new observations and clinical correlation. AJR Am J Roentgenol 1998;171(3):713–6.

[37] Atta MG, Longenecker JC, Fine DM, et al. Sonography as a predictor of human immunodeficiency virus-associated nephropathy. J Ultrasound Med 2004;23(5):603–10.

[38] Hamper UM, Goldblum LE, Hutchins GM, et al. Renal involvement in AIDS: sonographic-pathologic correlation. AJR Am J Roentgenol 1988; 150(6):1321–5.

RADIOLOGIC CLINICS OF NORTH AMERICA

Radiol Clin N Am 44 (2006) 777–786

Sonography of Benign Renal Cystic Disease

Therese M. Weber, MD

- Simple cortical cysts
- Complex renal cysts
- Renal sinus cysts
- Medullary cystic disease
- Multiple renal cysts
- Autosomal dominant polycystic kidney disease
- Autosomal recessive polycystic kidney disease
- Von Hippel-Lindau disease
- Tuberous sclerosis
- Acquired cystic kidney disease associated with dialysis
- Multiloculated cystic renal masses
- Multicystic dysplastic kidney
- Multilocular cystic nephroma
- Summary
- Acknowledgments
- References

When evaluating renal masses, differentiating cysts from solid lesions is the primary role of ultrasound (US). US is also helpful and frequently superior to CT, in demonstrating the complex internal architecture of cystic lesions in terms of internal fluid content, septations, tiny nodules, and wall abnormalities, including associated soft tissue masses. Renal cysts are common in the population older than 50 years, occurring in at least 50% of people [1]. Scanning technique is important to the success of demonstrating renal masses with US. The kidneys should be evaluated in multiple patient positions, including supine, lateral decubitus, and occasionally oblique or prone positions. The mass should be scanned with an appropriate focal zone. Simple renal cysts will frequently be better demonstrated with tissue harmonic imaging, which can eliminate low-level internal echoes by reducing background noise [2]. The Bosniak Classification System of renal cysts, shown in Box 1, has become an important tool used by radiologists and urologists to communicate the significance of renal cyst imaging characteristics [3,4]. The primary goal of the radiologist in evaluating cystic renal masses is the differentiation of nonsurgical from surgical lesions [5].

Simple cortical cysts

The sonographic criteria used to diagnose a simple cyst include the following characteristics: internally anechoic, posterior acoustic enhancement, and a sharply defined, imperceptible, smooth far wall. Simple cysts are usually round or ovoid in shape. If all these sonographic criteria are met, further evaluation or follow-up is not required. Maintaining rigid criteria is necessary to ensure the highest possible accuracy with US [6]. The simple renal cyst is a Bosniak category I cyst [Fig. 1] [3].

Complex renal cysts

Complex cysts do not meet the strict US criteria of a simple renal cyst. Five to ten percent of all renal

This article was originally published in *Ultrasound Clinics* 1:1, January 2006.
Department of Radiology, Wake Forest University School of Medicine, Medical Center Boulevard, Winston-Salem, NC 27157-1088, USA
E-mail address: tweber@wfubmc.edu

doi:10.1016/j.rcl.2006.10.013

Box 1: Bosniak classification of renal cystic disease

Category I

Simple benign cyst by imaging criteria

Category II

Cystic lesions characterized by:

- One or two thin (≤1 mm thick) septations or thin, fine calcification in the wall or septa
- Hyperdense, homogeneous benign cysts
- Diameter of 3 cm or less
- One quarter of its wall extending outside the kidney so the wall can be assessed
- No contrast enhancement

Category IIF

Cystic lesions that are minimally complicated that need follow-up. Some suspicious features in these lesions need follow-up to detect any change in character.

Category III

True indeterminate cystic masses that need surgical evaluation, although many prove to be benign, characterized by:

- Uniform wall thickening or nodularity
- Thick or irregular peripheral calcification
- Multilocular nature with multiple enhancing septa
- Hyperdense lesions that do not meet category II criteria

Category IV

Lesions with findings that are clearly malignant, including:

- Nonuniform or enhancing thick wall
- Enhancing or large nodules in the wall
- Clearly solid components in the cystic lesions
- Irregular margins

Size criterion of 3 cm differentiates between II and IIF lesions. These cysts need at least 6-month follow-up and are most likely benign but somewhat suspicious [8]. Many of these cysts, depending on the degree of abnormality, will require further imaging with MR or CT.

Internal echoes within a renal cyst may be caused by a complicating hemorrhage or infection. Infected cysts on US usually have a thickened wall and may exhibit a debris-fluid or gas-fluid level. Aspiration and drainage may be required for diagnosis and treatment. Hemorrhagic cysts can usually be followed with serial US examination if there is no evidence of malignancy at MR or CT evaluation. Septations within a cyst may occur following hemorrhage, infection, or percutaneous aspiration [Fig. 2]. Two adjacent cysts may share a common wall and mimic a large septated cyst. There may be a small amount of renal parenchyma between two adjacent cysts, suggesting a thick septation. If septa are "paper" thin (≤1 mm), smooth, and attached to the cyst wall without focal thickening or nodularity, a benign cyst can be diagnosed [3,8]. Fewer than five septations should be present in a benign cyst. If the cystic lesion shows septal irregularity, septal thickness greater than 1 mm, thick calcifications, or solid elements at the wall attachment, the lesion must be presumed malignant and requires further evaluation with MR or CT.

Calcifications in renal cysts may be fine and linear, or amorphous and thick. The presence of a small amount of calcium or thin, fine areas of calcification in the wall or a septation, without an associated soft tissue nodule, likely represents a complicated cyst rather than malignancy. Thick, irregular, amorphous calcification had been thought to be more concerning for malignancy; however, a recent report demonstrates that calcification in a cystic renal mass is not as important in the diagnosis as the presence of enhancing soft-tissue elements [9]. Renal cysts with milk-of-calcium will show layering, echogenic, dependent material that may be mobile. These cysts are always benign. At real-time US, bright echogenic foci with ringdown may be seen on septa and in the cyst walls; however, calcification may not be of sufficient density to be identified on CT examination.

Bosniak category III lesions are moderately complicated cysts that have more numerous or thickened septae; a thickened wall; thicker, irregular calcification; or multiloculated features. Benign and malignant tumors may be classified as Bosniak category III lesions. Because most category III lesions will be malignant [10], all category III lesions require surgical resection or biopsy. Benign lesions in this category include the multilocular cystic nephroma; complex septated and multiloculated

cysts are not simple cysts, and 5% to 10% of renal cysts with complex features prove to be tumors [7]. These complex renal cysts may contain complex fluid, septations, calcification, perceptible defined wall, or mural nodularity. Bosniak category II cysts are minimally complicated cysts that may contain septations or thin calcification, and include infected cysts and high-density cysts seen on noncontrast CT examination. High-density cysts are defined as having a density greater than 20 Hounsfield units (HU) on noncontrast CT. US may confirm the cystic nature in 50% of these lesions, especially if larger in size (1.5–3.0 cm). Equivocal cases can be placed in category IIF, created for minimally complicated cysts that require follow-up.

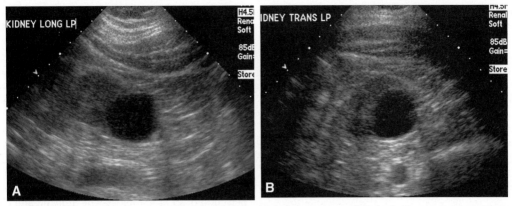

Fig. 1. Simple cyst in the lower renal pole in longitudinal (*A*) and transverse (*B*) planes demonstrating character-istic sonographic findings.

cysts; densely calcified cysts; a complex abscess; an infected cyst; vascular malformation; xanthogranu-lomatous pyelonephritis (XGP); or echinococcosis. Malignant lesions in this category include cystic Wilms' tumor in a child and cystic adenocarcinoma in an adult. Bosniak category IV lesions are cystic or necrotic carcinomas that may have solid elements, irregular margins, and enhancement demonstrated on CT, MRI, or US with contrast imaging. These le-sions are unequivocally malignant and require treatment. Renal cystic lesions with perceptible, de-fined, thickened wall; thick septae; mural nodular-ity; intracystic soft tissue mass; or abnormal calcifications on US are concerning for malignancy.

Renal sinus cysts

Renal sinus cysts (RSCs) are common and have been described as peripelvic cysts, parapelvic lym-phatic cysts, parapelvic lymphangiectasia, and para-pelvic cysts [11]. RSCs are likely lymphatic in origin or develop from embryologic rests. These cysts do not communicate with the collecting system [12]. Most RSCs are asymptomatic, but they may become

infected or bleed, and may cause hematuria, hyper-tension, or hydronephrosis [13]. There are two dis-tinct patterns of cyst formation in the renal sinus that include multiple, small, confluent cysts versus a single, larger cyst that probably arises from the ad-jacent parenchyma [11]. On US, these are simple cysts located in the medullary or renal sinus area of the kidney. Multiple renal sinus cysts mimic hy-dronephrosis on US and noncontrasted CT. If com-munication with the collecting system cannot be demonstrated with US to confirm hydronephrosis, additional studies such as intravenous pyelogram, contrasted CT, or MR examination may be needed.

Medullary cystic disease

Medullary cystic disease is a group of similar dis-eases that occur as a result of progressive renal tubu-lar atrophy with secondary glomerular sclerosis and medullary cystic formation [14,15]. Medullary cys-tic disease is an important cause of end-stage renal disease (ESRD) in children, accounting for 10% to 25% of the cases of ESRD. Two distinct presenta-tions occur. The childhood form, which is most

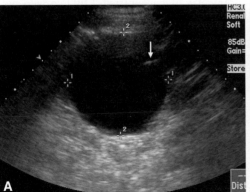
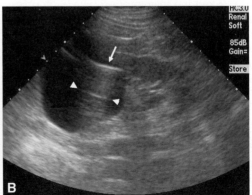

Fig. 2. (*A*) Mildly complicated renal cyst with thin septation (*white arrow*). (*B*) Artifact (*white arrowheads*) from the septation is frequently seen at real-time sonography.

common, is inherited as an autosomal recessive disorder. There is an association with extrarenal, ophthalmologic abnormalities. The adult form, inherited as an autosomal dominant pattern, tends to present in early adulthood and is not associated with extrarenal abnormalities. US findings include kidneys that are small to normal in size, are hyperechoic, and have small (0.1 to 1.0 cm) cysts in the medulla and at the corticomedullary junction [16,17]. Acquired cystic kidney disease may resemble medullary cystic disease; however, cyst location in the cortex and a history of dialysis supports the diagnosis of acquired cystic kidney disease.

Multiple renal cysts

With increased use of CT, US, and MR, patients who are harboring multiple simple cysts or lesions too small to characterize are being seen with increasing frequency. Multiple renal cysts can be seen in polycystic kidney disease, Von Hippel-Lindau disease (VHL), tuberous sclerosis (TS), acquired cystic kidney disease associated with dialysis (ACKDD), and mulitcystic dysplastic kidney.

Autosomal dominant polycystic kidney disease

Autosomal dominant polycystic kidney disease (ADPKD) is the third most common systemic hereditary condition and accounts for 10% to 15% of all patients on dialysis [18]. Because the disease is characterized by variable expression and occurs with spontaneous mutation, up to 50% of patients will have no family history of the disease [19]. Renal failure develops in 50% of patients and is usually present by 60 years of age. Early signs of the disease include hypertension and flank or back pain with variable progression to ESRD. Nephrolithiasis occurs in 20% to 36% of patients because of metabolic (lower glomerular filtration rate and urine volume) and anatomic (associated with larger and more numerous renal cysts) factors [20]. Extrarenal manifestations of ADPKD include hepatic, pancreatic, ovarian, splenic, arachnoid, and other cysts, and intracranial berry aneurysms with associated intracranial hemorrhage, abdominal aortic aneurysm, cardiac valve abnormalities, and hernias. The vascular abnormalities and cyst development are related to a basement membrane defect [18]. Eighty percent of people who have ADPKD and ESRD will have colonic diverticulosis. At least two different genes involving chromosomes 4 and 16 have been found to be associated with ADPKD [21].

US, because of high sensitivity and low cost, has become the primary method of diagnosing ADPKD and following the cysts. US screening for ADPKD typically begins between ages 10 and 15 years, but has the problem of false negatives in about 14% of patients younger than 30 years. Bear and colleagues [22] developed criteria that are widely used to diagnose ADPKD. In adults who have a family history of ADPKD, the presence of at least three cysts in both kidneys, with at least one cyst in each kidney, is a positive finding [23]. The cysts tend to involve all portions of the kidney and are of variable size. US typically reveals kidneys that are bilaterally enlarged with compression of the central sinus echo complex [Fig. 3]. When the kidneys are markedly enlarged with multiple complex cysts, detection of solid lesions may be difficult, and correlation with MR may be necessary to evaluate for renal cell carcinoma (RCC). When a solid mass is seen it can be confirmed with confidence sonographically [Fig. 4]. Nephrolithiasis may be difficult to demonstrate sonographically because of distortion of the collecting system by numerous large cysts. There is no increased risk for RCC in patients who have ADPKD, except for increased risk related to dialysis and the generally increased risk for RCC in men.

Autosomal recessive polycystic kidney disease

Autosomal recessive polycystic kidney disease (ARPKD) is characterized by varying degrees of renal failure and portal hypertension as a result of dilatation of renal collecting tubules, dilatation of biliary radicals, and periportal fibrosis that influences its presentation. The involved gene is located on chromosome 6 [24]. In its severest form, renal disease predominates and ARPKD manifests itself immediately after birth with the early complication of severe pulmonary failure. The diagnosis may be made at fetal or neonatal US. Characteristically, the kidneys are enlarged bilaterally, and oligohydramnios, Potter's facies, and pulmonary complications may be encountered. Children who present later will have some element of renal impairment with the complications of congenital hepatic fibrosis, including portal hypertension, splenomegaly, and bleeding varices [25]. With US, the kidneys maintain a reniform shape, but may be normal to bilaterally enlarged and echogenic [Fig. 5].

Von Hippel-Lindau disease

VHL disease is an uncommon condition characterized by multiple lesions, including hemangioblastomas in the central nervous system (CNS) and retina; RCC; pheochromocytomas; pancreatic neuroendocrine tumors; epididymal cystadenomas; endolymphatic sac tumors; carcinoid tumors; and

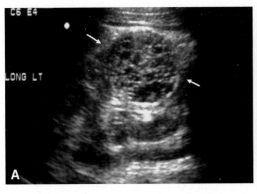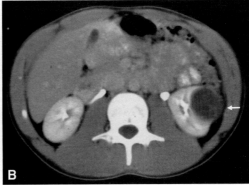

Fig. 9. Longitudinal US (*A*) and CT (*B*) images demonstrating a predominantly cystic mass with multiple internal septations, proven at surgery to be a multilocular cystic nephroma. Note the better representation of the lesion's internal architecture at US.

eighth decades. MLCN consists of multiple epithelially lined cysts that do not communicate. MLCN is usually a benign neoplasm; however, metastases have been reported [5,39]. US will show a mass containing multiple cysts or internal septations [Fig. 9]. It is not possible to conclusively distinguish MLCN from multiloculated RCC radiolographically, and these are usually surgical lesions.

Summary

US plays an important role in evaluation of the kidney in cases of medical renal disease because of lower cost, ready availability, lack of radiation, and lack of need for iodinated contrast material. The primary role of US in evaluating benign cystic renal disease is the distinction of a simple cyst from a solid mass, and in defining the characteristics of a complex cyst.

Acknowledgments

The author would like to acknowledge Raymond B. Dyer, MD, for his editorial assistance.

References

[1] Kissane JM. Congenital malformations. In: Hepinstall RH, editor. Pathology of the kidney. Boston: Little, Brown; 1973. p. 69–119.

[2] Schmidt T, Holh C, Haage P, et al. Diagnostic accuracy of phase-inversion tissue harmonic imaging versus fundamental B-mode sonography in the evaluation of focal lesions of the kidney. AJR Am J Roentgenol 2003;180:1639–47.

[3] Bosniak MA. The current radiological approach to renal cysts. Radiology 1986;158:1–10.

[4] Leder RA. Radiological approach to renal cysts and the Bosniak classification system. Curr Opin Urol 1999;9(2):129–33.

[5] Hartman DS, Choyke PL, Hartman MS. A practical approach to the cystic renal mass. Radiographics 2004;24:S101–15.

[6] Bosniak MA. The small (<3 cm) renal parenchymal tumor: detection, diagnosis, and controversies. Radiology 1991;179:307–17.

[7] Zeman RK, Cronan JJ, Rosenfield AT, et al. Imaging approach to the suspected renal mass. Radiol Clin North Am 1985;23(3):503–29.

[8] Israel GM, Bosniak MA. Follow-up CT of moderately complex cystic lesions of the kidney (Bosniak category IIF). AJR Am J Roentgenol 2003; 181:627–33.

[9] Israel GM, Bosniak MA. Calcification in cystic renal masses: is it important in diagnosis? Radiology 2003;226:47–52.

[10] Harisingani MG, Maher MM, Gervais DA, et al. Incidence of malignancy in complex cystic renal masses (Bosniak category III): should imaging-guided biopsy precede surgery? AJR Am J Roentgenol 2003;180:755–8.

[11] Rha SE, Byun JY, Jung SE, et al. The renal sinus: pathologic spectrum and multimodality imaging approach. Radiographics 2004;24:S117–31.

[12] Hidalgo H, Dunnick NR, Rosenburg ER, et al. Parapelvic cysts: appearance on CT and sonography. AJR Am J Roentgenol 1982;138:667–71.

[13] Chan JCM, Kodroff MB. Hypertension and hematuria secondary to parapelvic cyst. Pediatrics 1980;65:821–3.

[14] Gardner KD. Juvenile nephronophthiasis and renal medullary cystic disease. In: Gardner KD, editor. Cystic disease of the kidney. New York: John Wiley & Sons; 1976. p. 173–85.

[15] Wise SW, Hartman DS. Medullary cystic disease of the kidney. In: Pollack HM, McClennan BL, editors. Clinical urography: an atlas and textbook of urologic imaging. 2nd edition. Philadelphia: W.B. Saunders Company; 2000. p. 1398–403.

[16] Resnick JS, Hartman DS. Medullary cystic disease of the kidney. In: Polack HM, editor. Clinical urology: an atlas and textbook of urologic

imaging. Philadelphia: W.B. Saunders Company; 1990. p. 1178–84.

[17] Rego JD, Laing FG, Jeffrey RB. Ultrasonic diagnosis of medullary cystic disease. J Ultrasound Med 1983;2:433–6.

[18] Choyke PL. Inherited cystic diseases of the kidney. Radiol Clin North Am 1996;34(5):925–46.

[19] Dalgaard OZ. Bilateral polycystic disease of the kidney: A follow-up of 284 patients and their families. Acta Med Scand 1957;157(S328):1–255.

[20] Grampsas SA, Chandhoke PS, Fan J, et al. Anatomic and metabolic risk factors for nephrolithiasis in patients with autosomal dominant polycystic kidney disease. Am J Kidney Dis 2000;36(1):53–7.

[21] Fick GM, Gabow PA. Natural history of autosomal dominant polycystic kidney disease. Annu Rev Med 1994;45:23–9.

[22] Bear JC, McManamon P, Morgan J, et al. Age at clinical onset and at ultrasound detection of adult polycystic kidney disease. Data for genetic counseling. Am J Med Genet 1984;18:45–53.

[23] Parfrey PS, Bear JC, Morgan J, et al. The diagnosis and prognosis of autosomal dominant polycystic kidney disease. N Engl J Med 1990;323:1085–90.

[24] Dimitrakov JD, Dimitrakov DI. Autosomal recessive polycystic kidney disease. Clinical and genetic profile. Folia Med (Plovdiv) 2003;45:5–7.

[25] Harris PC, Rosetti S. Molecular genetics of autosomal recessive polycystic kidney disease. Mol Genet Metab 2004;81:75–85.

[26] Sano T, Horiguchi H. Von Hippel-Lindau disease. Microsc Res Tech 2003;60:159–64.

[27] Kaelin WG Jr. The von Hippel-Lindau tumor suppressor gene and kidney cancer. Clin Cancer Res 2004;10:6290S–5S.

[28] Richard S, David P, Marsot-Dupuch K, et al. Central nervous system hemangioblastomas, endolymphatic sac tumors, and von Hippel-Lindau disease. Neurosurg Rev 2000;23:1–22.

[29] Gomez MR. Tuberous sclerosis. New York: Raven Press; 1988.

[30] Torres VE. Systemic manifestations of renal cystic disease. In: Gardner KD, Bernstein J, editors. The cystic kidney. Dordrecht (The Netherlands): Kluwer Academic Publishers; 1990. p. 207.

[31] Zimmerhackl LB, Rehm M, Kaufmehl K, et al. Renal involvement in tuberous sclerosis complex: a retrospective survey. Pediatr Nephrol 1994;8:451–7.

[32] Hildebrandt F. Genetic renal disease in children. Curr Opin Pediatr 1995;7:182–91.

[33] Dunnill MS, Millard PR, Oliver D. Acquired cystic kidney disease of the kidneys: a hazard of long-term intermittent maintenance haemodialysis. J Clin Pathol 1977;30:868–77.

[34] Levine E, Slusher SL, Grantham JJ, et al. Natural history of acquired cystic kidney disease in dialysis patients: a prospective longitudinal CT study. AJR Am J Roentgenol 1991;156:501–6.

[35] Port FK, Ragheb NE, Schwartz AG, et al. Neoplasms in dialysis patients: a population-bases study. Am J Kidney Dis 1989;14:119–23.

[36] Matson MA, Cohen EP. Acquired cystic kidney disease: occurrence, prevalence, and renal cancers. Medicine 1990;69:217–26.

[37] Allan PL. Ultrasonography of the native kidney in dialysis and transplant patients. J Clin Ultrasound 1992;20:557–67.

[38] Strife JF, Souza AS, Kirks DR, et al. Multicystic Dysplastic kidney in children: US follow-up. Radiology 1993;186:785–8.

[39] Madewell JE, Goldman SM, Davis CJ, et al. Multilocular cystic nephroma: a radiographic-pathologic correlation of 58 patients. Radiology 1983;146:309–21.

RADIOLOGIC
CLINICS
OF NORTH AMERICA

Radiol Clin N Am 44 (2006) 787–803

ELSEVIER
SAUNDERS

Sonography in Benign and Malignant Renal Masses

Raj Mohan Paspulati, MD[a],*, Shweta Bhatt, MD[b]

Ultrasonography is often the initial modality for imaging of the kidneys, although contrast-enhanced CT is the established imaging modality for the diagnosis of renal tumors. Despite technical limitations, a large percentage of renal tumors can be characterized by ultrasonography. Cystic and solid renal parenchymal mass lesions can be well differentiated by ultrasonography. Technical advances in the gray-scale and color-flow Doppler (CFD) ultrasound have improved the sensitivity in detection of small renal tumors. Gray-scale and CFD ultrasonography can demonstrate the vascular invasion in selected groups of patients who have renal cell carcinoma (RCC). Contrast-enhanced Doppler ultrasonography appears promising as a cost-effective, noninvasive imaging technique in the characterization and follow-up of indeterminate renal mass lesions. As nephron-sparing surgery is being increasingly used in the management of small RCC, intraoperative ultrasound (US) has become a useful tool in guiding the surgeon. This article reviews the gray-scale and CFD features of benign and malignant renal masses encountered in radiology practice.

This article was originally published in *Ultrasound Clinics* 1:1, January 2006.

[a] Department of Radiology, University Hospitals of Cleveland, Case Western Reserve University, 11100 Euclid Avenue, Cleveland, OH 44106, USA

[b] Department of Radiology, University of Rochester Medical Center, 601 Elmwood Avenue, Box 648, Rochester, NY 14642, USA

* Corresponding author.
E-mail address: paspulati@uhrad.com (R.M. Paspulati).

doi:10.1016/j.rcl.2006.10.002

Normal sonographic anatomy of the kidney

The kidneys are bean-shaped retroperitoneal organs with their medial aspects parallel to the lateral margin of the adjacent psoas muscles. The normal orientation of the kidneys is such that the upper pole is medial and anterior to the lower pole. The right kidney is 1 to 2 cm inferior in position as compared with the left kidney because of the location of the liver superior to the right kidney. The renal size varies with the age, sex, and body habitus. The measurement of renal volume is a more effective way of assessing the renal size, though measurement of renal length is more practical in regular practice [1]. The normal adult kidney measures 10 to 12 cm in length, 4 to 5 cm in width, and 2.5 to 3 cm in thickness. A discrepancy of more than 2 cm between the lengths of two kidneys is considered significant and needs further evaluation. The liver and hepatic flexure of the colon are situated anterior to the right kidney. The spleen lies anterosuperior to the left kidney and the rest of the left kidney is related anteriorly with the colon.

On ultrasonography of a normal kidney, there is good differentiation of the renal capsule, cortex, medulla, and central sinus complex [Fig. 1]. The renal capsule is visible as an echogenic line because of the interface between the echogenic perinephric fat and renal cortex. The renal parenchyma is composed of outer cortex and inner medulla (pyramids). The renal cortex is echogenic as compared with the medulla, but is iso- to hypoechoic as compared with the normal hepatic or splenic parenchyma. The extension of renal cortex toward the renal sinus between the renal pyramids forms the columns of Bertin. The central sinus is composed of fat, fibrous tissue, renal vessels, and lymphatic vessels. It has highest echogenicity because of the adipose tissue, and its size increases with the age of the person.

Sonographic technique

Sonographic evaluation of the right kidney is ideally performed from an anterior oblique approach

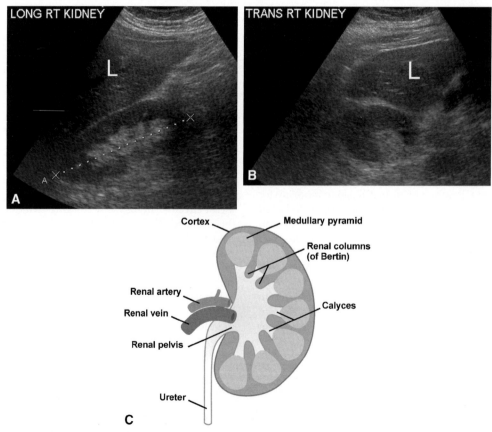

Fig. 1. Normal kidney. Longitudinal (*A*) and transverse (*B*) gray-scale US of the normal right kidney (calipers show the maximum longitudinal dimension of the kidney). (*C*) The schematic representation of the sagittal section of the kidney. L, liver.

using liver as an acoustic window, whereas the left kidney is scanned through a posterior oblique approach. The lower pole of the right kidney may be imaged using a more posterior approach. The upper pole of the left kidney is often best seen through an intercostal approach using spleen as a window. In addition to supine position, decubitus, prone, or upright positions may provide better images of the kidneys [2]. An appropriate transducer frequency ranging from 2.5 to 5 MHz should be used, depending on the body habitus. Time gain compensation and adjustment of other scanning parameters will allow a uniform acoustic pattern throughout the image [3]. Renal echogenicity should be compared with the echogenicity of the liver and spleen [2]. The renal parenchyma of a normal adult kidney is hypoechoic to the liver and spleen. The sonographic examination of the kidneys should include long axis and transverse views of the upper poles, midportions, and the lower poles, with assessment of the cortex and central sinus. Maximum measurement of renal length should be recorded for both kidneys [2]. Kidneys and the perirenal regions should be assessed for abnormalities. CFD and Power Doppler (PD) are used to differentiate vascular from nonvascular structures.

Pseudolesions of kidney

There are various developmental variants of the kidney that need to be identified on sonography to avoid misdiagnosis as renal neoplasm or other renal pathology [Table 1].

Dromedary hump

Dromedary hump is a common renal variation usually seen as a focal bulge on the lateral border of the left kidney [Fig. 2]. It is a result of adaptation of the

renal surface to the adjacent spleen. It can be easily differentiated from a renal mass because of its similar echotexture to that of adjacent renal parenchyma on gray-scale ultrasound. CFD and PD will demonstrate similar perfusion to that of adjacent renal parenchyma.

Persistent fetal lobulation

Persistent fetal lobulation is another common renal variant that can be mistaken for renal scarring, a consequence of chronic infective process of the kidneys. Persistent fetal lobulation can be differentiated from scarred kidneys by the location of the renal surface indentations, which do not overlie the medullary pyramids as in true renal scarring [4], but overlie the space between the pyramids [Fig. 3]. The underlying medulla and the cortex are normal.

Prominent column of Bertin (hypertrophy)

Prominent column of Bertin is a prominent cortical tissue that is present between the pyramids and projects into the renal sinus [Fig. 4]. If not identified as a normal variant, it may be mistaken for an intrarenal tumor. Sonography can accurately identify it by depicting its continuity with the renal cortex and a similar echo pattern as the renal parenchyma. CFD and PD imaging can further assist by depicting a similar vascular pattern as that of normal renal tissue [5,6]. Prominent columns of Bertin are usually seen in the middle third of the kidney and are more common on the left side [5].

Junctional parenchymal defect

Junctional parenchymal defect (JPD) is another variant commonly mistaken for a cortical scar or a hyperechogenic renal tumor. JPD is a linear or triangular hyperechoic structure in the anterosuperior or posteroinferior surface of the kidney [Fig. 5].

Table 1: Renal pseudotumors

Pseudotumor	Diagnostic imaging features
Congenital normal variants	
Dromedary hump	Focal bulge in the lateral contour of left kidney with echotexture similar to renal parenchyma
Persistent fetal lobulation	Renal surface indentations overlying the space between the pyramids
Prominent column of Bertin	Continuity with the normal cortex; echotexture and vascular perfusion similar to the normal cortex
Junctional parenchymal defect	Characteristic location in the anterosuperior and posteroinferior surface of the kidney and demonstration of continuity with the central sinus
Hypoechoic renal sinus fat	No distinct margin and normal vessels traversing the sinus
Inflammatory lesions	Diagnosis is based on the proper clinical context
Focal bacterial nephritis	
Renal abscess	

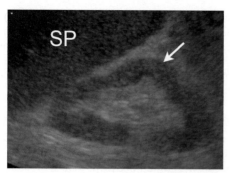

Fig. 2. Dromedary hump. Longitudinal gray-scale sonogram of the left kidney demonstrates the dromedary hump (*arrow*). SP, spleen.

These are caused by normal extensions of the renal sinus at the junction of the embryonic renunculi. These are differentiated from pathologic lesions by their characteristic location and demonstrate continuity with the central sinus by an echogenic line called interrenicular septum [7–9].

Hypoechoic renal sinus

The echogenicity of the renal sinus may vary from echogenic to anechoic. Hypoechoic renal sinus may mimic a mass lesion [10]. Absence of a well-defined margin and demonstration of normal vessels traversing the renal sinus by CFD will aid in differentiating a hypoechoic renal sinus from a mass lesion [10].

Inflammatory mass lesions

Acute focal bacterial nephritis and renal abscess may present as renal mass lesions indistinguishable from a renal tumor by ultrasonography and contrast-enhanced CT. The clinical presentation will aid in

differentiating these inflammatory pseudotumors from RCC [11–13].

Benign renal tumors

Angiomyolipoma

Angiomyolipoma (AML) is a hamartoma and has variable amounts of mature adipose tissue, smooth muscle, and thick-walled blood vessels. Eighty percent of the AMLs are sporadic in occurrence and 20% of them are associated with tuberous sclerosis (TS). Presence of subependymal nodules and giant cell astrocytoma are sine qua non of TS, but not AML. On the contrary, 80% of the patients who have TS develop AMLs [14,15]. Patients who have TS develop AMLs at a much younger age, and these tend to be multiple, bilateral, and larger than in sporadic cases. AMLs in patients who have TS are more likely to grow and become symptomatic [15,16]. The presence of estrogen and progesterone receptors in angiolipomas has been reported, and such AMLs are more common in women and in TS. These AMLs tend to grow during pregnancy and present with hemorrhage [17,18]. Small AMLs are asymptomatic and are incidental findings on imaging. AMLs smaller than 4 cm are symptomatic and are at increased risk for spontaneous hemorrhage [16,19]. Massive retroperitoneal hemorrhage from AML, also known as Wunderlich's syndrome, has been found in 10% of patients.

The characteristic sonographic appearance of AML is a well-defined hyperechoic mass [Fig. 6]. This increased echogenicity is attributed to the fat content, multiple interfaces, heterogeneous cellular architecture, and multiple vessels within the tumor [20,21]. However, there is significant overlap between the imaging features of AML and RCC. Small

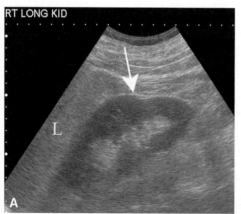

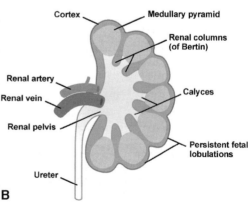

Fig. 3. Persistent fetal lobulations. Longitudinal (*A*) gray-scale sonogram of the right kidney demonstrates persistent fetal lobulation (*arrow*). L, liver. Schematic (*B*) appearance of persistent fetal lobulations (note fetal lobulations may be single or multiple).

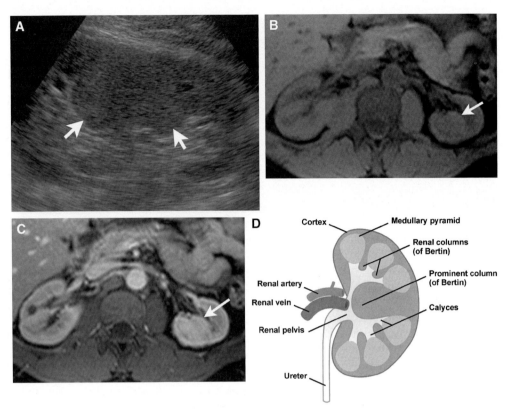

Fig. 4. Prominent column of Bertin. (*A*) Longitudinal gray-scale US of the left kidney demonstrates a prominent column of Bertin (*arrows*) mimicking an isoechoic renal mass. MRI was performed to confirm ultrasound findings. T1 flash fat-sat (*B*) and gadolinium-enhanced (*C*) MRI images of the kidneys reveal a prominent column of Bertin (*arrows*) seen in continuity with the renal cortex. (*D*) Schematic drawing of a prominent column of Bertin.

RCCs can be hyperechoic and indistinguishable from an AML on sonography. Acoustic shadowing, hypoechoic rim, and intratumoral cystic changes are some of the sonographic features found to be helpful in differentiating an AML from RCC. Hypoechoic rim and intratumoral cystic changes are seen only in RCC, whereas acoustic shadowing is observed with AML [Fig. 7] [22–24]. PD of AML may reveal focal intratumoral flow and a penetrating flow pattern [25]. The demonstration of intratumoral fat on CT confirms the diagnosis of an AML. The CT appearance of an AML also depends on the relative proportion of smooth muscle and vascular components of the tumor. Rarely, RCCs

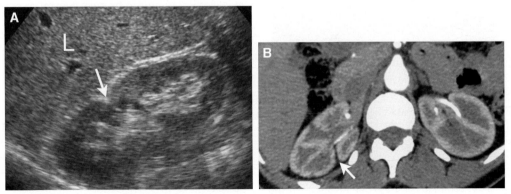

Fig. 5. Junctional parenchymal defect. (*A*) Longitudinal gray-scale US of the right kidney demonstrates a notch in the lateral border (*arrow*). L, liver. (*B*) Contrast-enhanced CT of the kidneys in another patient demonstrates the junctional parencymal defect (*arrow*).

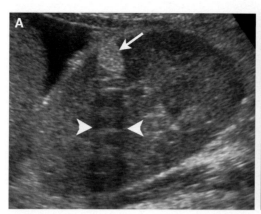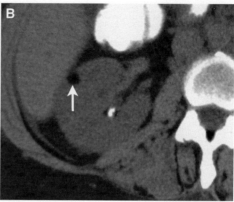

Fig. 6. Angiomyolipoma. (A) Longitudinal gray-scale US of the right kidney demonstrates an echogenic mass (*arrow*) with posterior acoustic shadowing (*arrowheads*). (B) Corresponding CT (excretory phase) confirms this lesion to be an angiomyolipoma, seen as a fat attenuation lesion (*arrow*) with a household unit of -8.

can demonstrate fat attenuation caused by entrapment of the perinal or renal sinus fat, lipid necrosis, or osseous metaplasia [26]. The characteristic intratumoral fat cannot be detected in 4.5% of AMLs, and will have high attenuation on an unenhanced CT scan. This finding has been attributed to minimal fat content or immature fat [25,27]. These AMLs with low fat content demonstrate homogeneous and prolonged enhancement on a contrast-enhanced scan, which distinguishes them from an RCC [25,28]. These AMLs with minimal fat are iso-echoic with renal parenchyma on sonography [25]. The demonstration of micro- or macroaneurysms at angiography is reported to be characteristic of an AML [29].

The risk for spontaneous rupture and hemorrhage of an AML is related to the tumor size and the size of microaneurysms. AMLs larger than 4 cm and those with microaneurysms larger than 5 mm are reported to be at increased risk for spontaneous rupture [16,30,31]. Management options of AMLs

include observation, embolization, and partial or total nephrectomy. Prophylactic transcatheter embolization of AMLs larger than 4 cm is reported to prevent tumor growth and spontaneous rupture [19,31,32]. Kothary and colleagues [33] have described a high recurrence rate of AMLs after embolization in patients who have TS, and recommend long-term surveillance of these patients following embolization.

Renal adenoma

Renal cell adenoma is considered to be a benign counterpart of RCC, though the true nature and potential of this tumor is a subject of much debate. The size criterion used by many pathologists in distinguishing an adenoma from RCC is based on the initial observation by Bell, that renal cortical glandular tumors of smaller than 3 cm rarely metastasize [34,35]. There are no histopathologic, histochemical, immunologic, or imaging characteristics that distinguish a benign adenoma from an RCC [36]. Most pathologists consider these small renal cortical tumors to be premalignant or potentially malignant and believe that tumor size is not a valid differentiating criterion [37]. The widespread use of US and CT has resulted in the incidental detection of these tumors.

Oncocytoma

Renal oncocytoma is a benign tumor of renal tubular origin (renal tubular epithelium is also called *oncocyte*). It has the male predominance and age incidence similar to RCC. They are asymptomatic and are discovered as incidental findings on imaging [38]. They are well-defined tumors of variable size and can be as large as 20 cm [35]. The preoperative differentiation of oncocytomas from RCC is invaluable, but is often difficult because of overlap

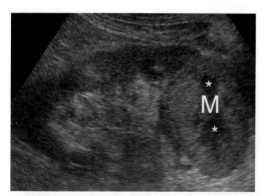

Fig. 7. RCC. Longitudinal gray-scale sonogram of the left kidney demonstrates a hyperechoic mass (M) arising from the lower pole with areas of intra tumoral cystic changes (*asterisk*).

of imaging features. The characteristic central stellate scar on cross-sectional imaging and spoke-wheel pattern of enhancement on an angiogram are infrequently seen in oncocytomas and can also be seen in RCC [39–41]. Oncocytomas can be hypoechoic, isoechoic, or hyperechoic to the renal parenchyma on sonography. MRI is reported to be superior to CT and US in identifying the imaging features of a small tumor [42]. The radiologic features, which are helpful in distinguishing an oncocytoma from RCC, include well-defined margins, homogeneous enhancement without hemorrhage, calcification or necrosis, presence of a central stellate scar, and spoke-wheel pattern of arterial enhancement. There are few reports of bilateral and multicentric oncocytomas [43,44]. Renal oncocytoma and RCC can coexist in the same or contralateral kidney [45,46]. Dechet and colleagues [47] have reported coexistent RCC in 10% of a total 138 cases of oncocytomas. Imaging-guided biopsy of renal tumors is indicated whenever there is radiologic suspicion of an oncocytoma [48–50].

Leiomyoma

Renal leiomyoma is a rare benign tumor of smooth muscle origin. These tumors are either peripheral, arising from the renal capsule, or central in parapelvic location. They are more common in women between the second and fifth decades of life. Most renal leiomyomas are asymptomatic, with incidental detection on routine diagnostic imaging. These are well-defined tumors and are indistinguishable from RCC by imaging. Renal leiomyomas have variable appearance on imaging: from that of an entirely solid, to a mixed solid/cystic, to an entirely cystic lesion. Renal leiomyomas appear as well-defined hypoechoic solid mass lesions on ultrasonography. The peripheral lesions may extend into the retroperitoneum and can resemble primary retroperitoneal sarcomas. The central lesions will have a mass effect over the collecting system and renal vasculature. They are most often avascular or hypovascular on angiogram [51–53].

Hemangioma

Hemangiomas are uncommon benign tumors of the kidney that can present with macroscopic hematuria. They are commonly located in the renal pyramids and renal pelvis, and are classified into capillary and cavernous hemangiomas. The vascular spaces are small in capillary hemangioma and large in cavernous hemangiomas. They are predominantly smaller than 1 cm, but occasionally present as large mass lesions [54]. Gray-scale US features a nonspecific solid mass, and CT demonstrates a well-defined low-density mass without significant enhancement [55,56]. Larger lesions may cause displacement of the renal vessels and collecting system. Angiography may demonstrate a hypovascular or hypervascular mass [57,58].

Juxtaglomerular tumor (reninoma)

Juxtaglomerular tumors are benign, renin-producing tumors of the kidney that arise from the afferent arterioles of the glomerulus. These tumors were first described by Robertson and colleagues in 1967 [59]. They are twice as common in women as in men. In a young patient who has hypertension, the presence of a renal mass, elevated serum renin levels, and hypokalemia should raise a suspicion of reninoma. The tumor is either hypo- or hyperechoic on sonography and appears as a well-defined hypodense solid mass on a contrast-enhanced CT. Angiography demonstrates a hypovascular mass with normal renal arteries. Renal vein sampling demonstrates elevated renin levels in reninomas, but renin is also elevated in renal artery stenosis. Surgical resection of the tumor results in reversal of hypertension and hypokalemia [60–62].

Hemangiopericytoma

Hemangiopericytomas are rare renal tumors with a malignant potential that arise from the pericytes. Tumor-induced hypoglycemia is characteristic of hemangiopericytoma and has been attributed to the production of insulin-like growth factors by the tumor. There are no distinguishing radiologic features of hemangiopericytoma from RCC or other mesenchymal tumors of the kidney [63–65].

Renal cell carcinoma

RCC is the most common primary malignancy of the kidney. It accounts for 2% of all malignancies. There has been a steady increase of 38% in the incidence of RCC between 1974 and 1990 [66]. The survival rates have also improved from 52% between 1974 and 1976 to 58% between 1983 and 1996 [66]. This trend has been attributed to the improved imaging technique and early diagnosis. Smith and colleagues [67] have reported that only 5.3% of the tumors between 1974 and 1977 were 3 cm or smaller as compared with 25.4% during 1982 to 1985. Of these small tumors in the later group, 96.7% were incidentally discovered by ultrasonography and CT. Most RCCs that are amenable for surgical cure by either partial nephrectomy or nephron-sparing surgery are incidentally detected by the increased use of cross-sectional imaging. Ultrasonography, being the primary imaging modality of the kidneys, is useful for screening and detection of small RCCs [68,69].

The RCCs are classified histologically into four main types [Table 2]. These include clear cell

Table 2: Classification of renal cell carcinoma

Subtype	Incidence	Grade	Imaging features
Clear (conventional) cell carcinoma	70%–80%	Low-grade tumor	Poor enhancement
Papillary type	10%–15%		
Type 1		Low-grade tumor	Poor enhancement
Type 2		Aggressive tumor	Intense enhancement
Chromophobe type	4%–5%	–	
Collecting duct type	<1%	Aggressive tumor with poor prognosis	–
Medullary carcinoma	<1%	Aggressive tumor with poor prognosis and common in sickle cell trait	–

carcinoma, papillary carcinoma, chromophobe carcinoma, and collecting duct carcinoma. The clear cell carcinomas are the most common type, accounting for 70% of the RCCs. The papillary type is the second most common type, accounting for 10% to 15% of the RCCs. The papillary type is subclasssified into type 1 and type 2 tumors. The type 2 papillary tumors are more aggressive than type 1. Clear cell and papillary tumors arise from the proximal tubular epithelium. The chromophobe carcinomas account for 5% of the RCCs and arise from cells of distal tubule. The collecting duct carcinomas are the least common type, arise from collecting duct epithelium, and are the most aggressive of all RCCs. The medullary carcinoma is a subtype of collecting duct carcinoma that is more common in patients who have sickle cell trait. Imaging cannot differentiate the different histologic types of RCC. The incidence of RCC is increased in acquired cystic disease of the kidney (ACDK). Clear cell carcinoma is the most common type of RCC associated with ACDK. The incidence of papillary type of RCC in ACDK is also higher than in the general population [70,71].

Hereditary renal cell carcinoma

RCCs are predominantly sporadic in occurrence and only 4% of them are familial in nature. The different types of hereditary RCCs are displayed in Table 3. The hereditary RCCs are characterized by autosomal dominant inheritance, presentation at a young age (third to fifth decades), and multifocal and bilateral tumors [72].

Clinical presentation of renal cell carcinoma

The classic clinical triad of hematuria, abdominal pain, and abdominal mass is seen in less than 10% of patients. About 20% to 40% present with paraneoplastic syndrome, which includes anemia, fever, hypertension, hypercalcemia, and hepatic dysfunction [73–75]. RCC can be associated with Stauffer syndrome, which is characterized by nonmetastatic intrahepatic cholestasis. This syndrome is a tumor-induced inflammatory response and is

Table 3: Hereditary renal cell carcinoma

Syndrome	Inheritance	Predominant renal tumor	Other renal lesions	Associated abnormalities
Von Hippel-Lindau	AD	Clear cell carcinoma	Cysts	Hemangioblastomas Retinal angiomas Pancreatic cysts Neuroendocrine tumors of pancreas Phaeochromocytoma
Hereditary papillary RCC	AD	Papillary type 1	None	None
Hereditary leiomyoma RCC	AD	Papillary type 2	None	Cutaneous and uterine leiomyomas
Birt-Hogg-Dubé	AD	Chromophobe carcinoma	Other types of RCC	Fibrofolliculomas Lung cysts Pneumothorax
Familial renal oncocytoma	–	Oncocytoma	None	–
Medullary carcinoma	–	Medullary carcinoma	None	Sickle cell trait

Abbreviation: AD, autosomal dominant.

reversible after resection of the tumor [76–78]. About 2% of the male patients present with left-sided varicocele because of renal vein involvement [79].

Imaging strategies of renal cell carcinoma

The goal of imaging is detection, diagnosis, and staging of RCC. Ultrasonography, CT, and MRI have variable sensitivity in detecting and staging RCC. Ultrasonography is less sensitive in detecting small renal lesions, especially those that do not deform the contour of the kidney. The sensitivity of CT and ultrasonography for detection of lesions 3 cm and less is 94% and 79%, respectively [80]. CT and MRI have nearly 100% accuracy in the diagnosis of RCC [81]. Ultrasonography is also less accurate than CT and MRI in staging of RCC. The accuracy of CT and MRI in staging of RCC ranges from 67% to 96%. Catalano and colleagues [82] have reported 96% sensitivity, 93% specificity, and 95% accuracy of multidetector CT (MDCT) in evaluating Robson stage I RCC. Robson and tumor, nodes, and metastases (TNM) staging of RCC are outlined in Table 4.

Despite these limitations, ultrasonography is still the initial imaging modality for screening and characterization of renal mass lesions. Ultrasonography is also useful in characterizing indeterminate renal mass lesions detected by CT, such as atypical cystic lesions, hypovascular solid mass lesions, and AMLs with minimal fat component [83].

Sonographic findings of renal cell carcinomas

The sonographic spectrum of RCCs varies from hypoechoic to hyperechoic solid mass lesions [Fig. 8]. RCCs 3 cm and smaller are predominantly hyperechoic and must be differentiated from AMLs [84,85]. The hyperechoic appearance is reported to be caused by papillary, tubular, or microcystic architecture; minute calcification; intratumoral hemorrhage; cystic degeneration; or fibrosis [24]. The presence of an anechoic rim caused by a pseudocapsule and intratumoral cystic changes can aid in differentiation of hyperechoic RCC from AML [24,86]. Several investigators have reported acoustic shadowing as a useful sign of AML [22,23]. Small isoechoic RCCs and those located at the poles can be missed by ultrasonography [26]. The isoechoic RCCs must be differentiated from pseudotumors, which include prominent column of Bertin, dromedary hump, persistent fetal lobulation, and compensatory hypertrophy. Careful attention to the morphology on gray-scale US will differentiate pseudotumors from a mass lesion. Power Doppler and contrast-enhanced sonography are useful in differentiating pseudotumors from true renal mass lesions by demonstrating similar vascularity of the pseudotumors to that of adjacent normal renal cortex [87,88]. Power Doppler and contrast-enhanced sonography will demonstrate the vascularity of a renal mass, but cannot differentiate an RCC from an AML [87,88].

Approximately 15% of the RCCs are cystic in nature and may result from extensive necrosis of a tumor, or represent a primary cystic renal carcinoma [89]. Histologically, the cystic RCCs are predominantly of clear cell type. RCCs with extensive necrosis are more aggressive as compared with the primary multilocular cystic RCCs [90,91]. Multilocular cystic RCC (MCRCC) is an uncommon subtype of RCC and constitutes about 3% of all RCCs. MCRCCs have a benign clinical course and may benefit from nephron-sparing surgery [92]. Cross-sectional imaging with US and CT of MCRCC will demonstrate well-defined, multilocular cystic mass with thin septations. Dystrophic calcification and mural nodules are less common and MCRCC should be included in the differential diagnosis of all multilocular cystic renal mass lesions in adults [93]. Small MCRCCs of less than 3 cm are hyperechoic on US and can mimic solid mass lesions, but show minimal enhancement on contrast-enhanced CT or MRI [94]. Contrast-enhanced Doppler US is reported to improve the diagnostic accuracy of malignant cystic renal mass by

Table 4: **Staging of renal cell carcinoma**

Robson stage	Tumor description	TNM stage
I	Tumor confined within renal capsule	
	Tumor <2.5 cm	T1
	Tumor >2.5 cm	T2
II	Tumor extension to perinephric fat or adrenal gland	T3a
III-A	Renal vein involvement or infradiaphragmatic IVC involvement	T3b
	Supradiaphragmatic IVC involvement	T3c
III-B	Regional lymph node metastases	N1–N3
III-C	Venous involvement and lymph node metastases	
IV-A	Invasion of adjacent organs beyond the Gerota's fascia	T4
IV-B	Distant metastases	

Abbreviations: IVC, inferior vena cava; TNM, tumor, nodes, metastases.

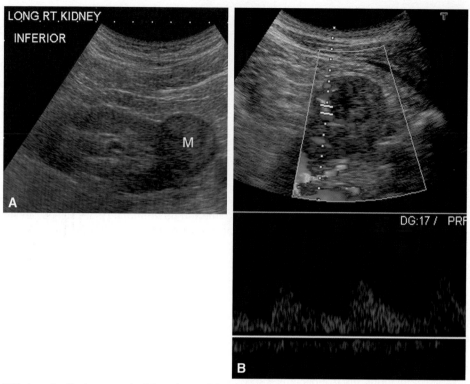

Fig. 8. RCC. Longitudinal gray-scale (*A*) and CFD (*B*) sonography of the right kidney demonstrates an iso- to hypoechoic mass arising from the lower pole, which shows presence of vascularity consistent with a RCC.

demonstrating the vascularity of the intracystic septations and mural nodules [95].

CT and MRI are the standard imaging methods for staging of RCC. However, US is useful in detecting the venous invasion and for demonstrating the cranial extent of the inferior vena cava (IVC) thrombus. Overall accuracy, sensitivity, and specificity of CFD for detecting the tumor involvement of renal vein and IVC is 93%, 81%, and 98%, respectively [96]. McGahan and colleagues [97] have reported a 100% sensitivity in the detection of renal vein involvement as compared with 89% sensitivity for IVC involvement by CFD sonography. Hence, US may be used as a complementary imaging modality when CT findings are equivocal in the assessment of venous extension of the tumor. The tumor thrombus is seen as an echogenic intraluminal mass causing distension of the vein. CFD will demonstrate flow around a bland thrombus and vascularity within a tumor thrombus. Use of US contrast agents is reported to improve the accuracy not only in demonstrating the extent of the thrombus but also in differentiating a tumor from a bland thrombus.

The prognosis of RCC will depend on the stage, histologic type, and grade of the tumor. The 5-year survival rates of TNM stages I, II, III, and IV are reported to be 91%, 74%, 67%, and 32%, respectively [98]. The presence of a sarcomatoid component is reported to have poor outcome [99].

Malignant uroepithelial tumors of the renal collecting system

Malignant uroepithelial tumors of the renal pelvis constitute about 5% of all the urinary tract neoplasms [100]. 90% of them are transitional cell carcinomas (TCC), 5% to 10% are squamous cell carcinomas, and less than 1% are adenocarcinomas [101,102].

Transitional carcinoma of renal pelvis

TCCs of the renal pelvis have similar epidemiologic features to those of bladder and ureter. The risk factors include exposure to chemicals in petroleum, rubber, and dye industries; analgesic abuse; and chronic inflammations. TCC is one of the several extracolonic manifestations of hereditary nonpolyposis colorectal cancer (HNPCC)/Lynch syndrome [103]. The mean age of presentation of TCC is 68 years with a higher rate of incidence in men than women. Painless hematuria is the characteristic clinical presentation of TCC [104]. Three morphologic forms of TCC are described, including focal intraluminal mass, mural thickening with narrowing of lumen, and an infiltrating mass in the renal sinus [105–107]. The excretory urogram has been the primary imaging modality for the diagnosis of TCC and is being replaced by CT or MR urogram [108,109]. These imaging modalities have the advantage of evaluating the entire urinary tract, which is crucial in the assessment of TCC.

Sonography demonstrates a poorly defined hypo- or hyperechoic mass in the renal sinus with or without pelvicaliectasis. The mass lesions are initially intraluminal and later invade the renal sinus fat and renal parenchyma. Infiltrating tumors of the renal parenchyma tend to preserve the reniform shape of the kidney [106,110].

Squamous cell carcinoma and adenocarcinoma

Squamous cell carcinoma is the second most common malignant uroepithelial tumor of the renal collecting system [Fig. 9]. Chronic irritation of the uroepithelium is the etiologic factor, which leads to squamous or columnar metaplasia of the transitional epithelium. Renal calculi with longstanding hydronephrosis and inflammation are important

predisposing factors for squamous cell carcinoma and adenocarcinoma of the renal pelvis [101,102,111]. The clinical presentation ranges from painless hematuria to nonspecific flank pain caused by hydronephrosis [101]. Squamous cell carcinomas are more aggressive than TCC and the tumor manifests as an infiltrating mass involving the collecting system, renal sinus fat, and renal parenchyma [112]. It is often difficult to differentiate squamous cell carcinoma of the renal pelvis from xanthogranulomatous pyelonephritis by imaging [113,114].

Renal metastases

The frequency of renal metastases is reported to vary from 7% to 13% based on autopsy findings [115,116]. More frequent use of cross-sectional imaging has resulted in an increase in the detection of renal metastases [117,118]. In patients who have a known history of malignancy, renal metastases are three times more common than primary renal tumors and are usually asymptomatic [115,116]. The tumors that most commonly metastasize to

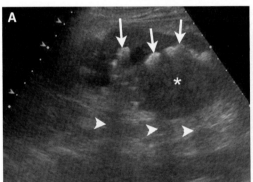
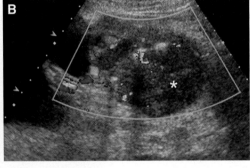
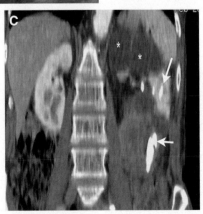

Fig. 9. Squamous cell carcinoma. Longitudinal gray-scale (*A*) and CFD (*B*) US of the left kidney demonstrates an enlarged kidney with areas of chunky calcification (*arrows*) with posterior acoustic shadowing (*arrowheads*). There is increased vascularity in the mass with large areas of necrosis (*asterisk*). Corresponding contrast-enhanced coronal CT (*C*) confirms the presence of calcification (*arrows*) and necrosis (*asterisk*). This tumor was pathologically confirmed to be a squamous cell carcinoma.

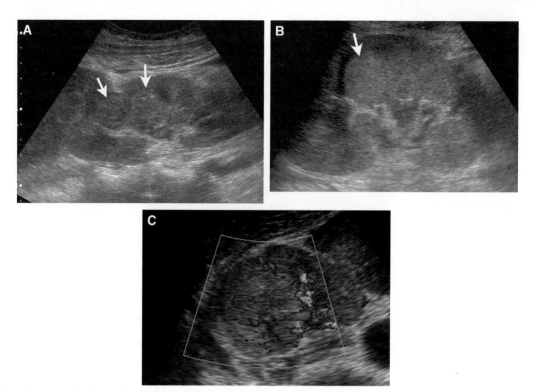

Fig. 10. Hyperechoic renal metastasis. Patient is a known case of esophageal carcinoma. Longitudinal gray-scale US of the right (*A*) and the left (*B*) kidney demonstrate multiple hyperechoic mass lesions (*arrows*). Tranverse CFD image (*C*) of the right kidney reveals increased vascularity.

the kidney are carcinoma of the lung, breast, and gastrointestinal tract, and melanoma [Fig. 10] [115,119]. The most common manifestation is bilateral, multiple renal mass lesions, though they can present with unilateral and solitary lesions. Renal metastases can be well-defined focal mass lesions or infiltrating in nature [117,120].

The most common sonographic appearance is hypoechoic, cortical mass lesions without through-transmission [Fig. 11] [121,122]. CT has higher sensitivity and accuracy than US in the detection of renal metastases [121–123]. In patients who have a known extrarenal primary malignancy, tissue sampling is necessary to differentiate metastases from a synchronous primary RCC [124].

Renal lymphoma

Renal lymphoma is commonly secondary to hematogeneous dissemination or contiguous extension from a retroperitoneal nodal disease. Primary lymphoma is rare as there is no lymphoid tissue in

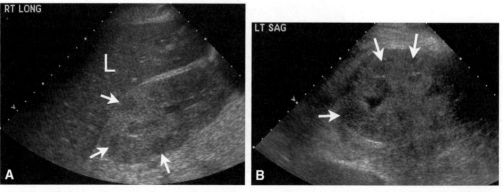

Fig. 11. Hypoechoic renal metastasis. Longitudinal gray-scale ultrasound of the right (*A*) and left (*B*) kidneys demonstrate multiple hypoechoic masses (*arrows*) in the renal parenchyma consistent with metastasis. L, liver.

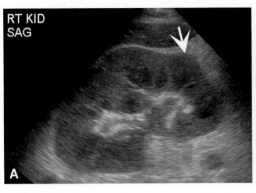 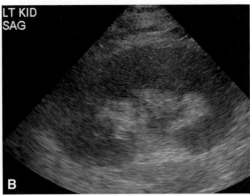

Fig. 12. Lymphoma. Longitudinal gray-scale US of the right (*A*) and the left (*B*) kidneys demonstrates bilaterally enlarged kidneys (R, 15.6 cm; L, 14.8 cm). In addition, right kidney also demonstrates a focal mass (*arrow*) in patient who has known non-Hodgkins lymphoma.

the kidney [125,126]. Though the reported incidence of renal involvement on autopsy ranges from 30% to 60%, the actual detection by imaging is only 3% to 8% [127]. The kidney is most commonly involved by the non-Hodgkin's B-cell type of lymphoma [128–130]. There is a wide spectrum of renal involvement of lymphoma. Unilateral or bilateral multiple renal mass lesions are the most common type of renal lymphoma. Bilateral renal involvement is reported to occur in 50% to 72% of lymphomas [Fig. 12]. Other manifestations include solitary renal mass, diffuse infiltration of the renal parenchyma, contiguous invasion from retroperitoneal disease, and isolated perinephric mass [127]. In the diffuse infiltrative form, there is proliferation of lymphoma within the interstitium of the renal parenchyma, resulting in enlarged kidneys with preservation of the reniform shape [120]. The renal mass lesions are homogenously hypoechoic on ultrasonography and are hypodense on a contrast-enhanced CT [120,131,132]. Spontaneous hemorrhage, cystic changes, and calcification are uncommon and are usually secondary to prior treatment [127].

Summary

CT is the gold standard for the detection and characterization of renal mass lesions and in staging of RCC. Despite its limitations, ultrasonography is often the first imaging modality of the kidneys and plays an important role in the diagnosis of renal tumors. Technical advances in the gray-scale ultrasonography have improved the detection of small RCCs. CFD and contrast-enhanced Doppler ultrasonography are useful in characterization of renal tumors and in the identification of pseudotumors.

As nephron-sparing surgery is now an established technique in the management of small RCC, intraoperative US has a key role in guiding the surgeon.

References

[1] Emamian SA, Nielsen MB, Pedersen JF, et al. Kidney dimensions at sonography: correlation with age, sex, and habitus in 665 adult volunteers. AJR Am J Roentgenol 1993;160:83–6.

[2] Grant EG, Barr LL, Borgstede J, et al. AIUM standard for the performance of an ultrasound examination of the abdomen or retroperitoneum. American Institute of Ultrasound in Medicine. J Ultrasound Med 2002;21:1182–7.

[3] Hagen-Ansert SL, Levzow B. Kidneys and adrenal glands. 3rd edition. St. Louis (MO): Mosby; 1993.

[4] Marchal G, Verbeken E, Oyen R, et al. Ultrasound of the normal kidney: a sonographic, anatomic and histologic correlation. Ultrasound Med Biol 1986;12:999–1009.

[5] Lafortune M, Constantin A, Breton G, et al. Sonography of the hypertrophied column of Bertin. AJR Am J Roentgenol 1986;146:53–6.

[6] Ascenti G, Zimbaro G, Mazziotti S, et al. Contrast- enhanced power Doppler US in the diagnosis of renal pseudotumors. Eur Radiol 2001; 11:2496–9.

[7] Tsushima Y, Sato N, Ishizaka H, et al. US findings of junctional parenchymal defect of the kidney. Nippon Igaku Hoshasen Gakkai Zasshi 1992;52:436–42.

[8] Carter AR, Horgan JG, Jennings TA, et al. The junctional parenchymal defect: a sonographic variant of renal anatomy. Radiology 1985;154: 499–502.

[9] Hoffer FA, Hanabergh AM, Teele RL. The interrenicular junction: a mimic of renal scarring on normal pediatric sonograms. AJR Am J Roentgenol 1985;145:1075–8.

[10] Seong CK, Kim SH, Lee JS, et al. Hypoechoic normal renal sinus and renal pelvis tumors: sonographic differentiation. J Ultrasound Med 2002;21:993-9 [quiz 1001-2].

[11] Schmidt H, Fischedick AR, Wiesmann W, et al. Acute focal bacterial nephritis. Rofo 1986;145: 245-9.

[12] Lee JK, McClennan BL, Melson GL, et al. Acute focal bacterial nephritis: emphasis on gray scale sonography and computed tomography. AJR Am J Roentgenol 1980;135:87-92.

[13] Soulen MC, Fishman EK, Goldman SM, et al. Bacterial renal infection: role of CT. Radiology 1989;171:703-7.

[14] Casper KA, Donnelly LF, Chen B, et al. Tuberous sclerosis complex: renal imaging findings. Radiology 2002;225:451-6.

[15] Ewalt DH, Sheffield E, Sparagana SP, et al. Renal lesion growth in children with tuberous sclerosis complex. J Urol 1991;160:141-5.

[16] Steiner MS, Goldman SM, Fishman EK, et al. The natural history of renal angiomyolipoma. J Urol 1993;150:1782-6.

[17] L'Hostis H, Deminiere C, Ferriere JM, et al. Renal angiomyolipoma: a clinicopathologic, immunohistochemical, and follow-up study of 46 cases. Am J Surg Pathol 1999;23:1011-20.

[18] Hatakeyama S, Habuchi T, Ichimura Y, et al. Rapidly growing renal angiomyolipoma during pregnancy with tumor thrombus into the inferior vena cava: a case report. Nippon Hinyokika Gakkai Zasshi 2002;93:48-51.

[19] Dickinson M, Ruckle H, Beaghler M, et al. Renal angiomyolipoma: optimal treatment based on size and symptoms. Clin Nephrol 1998;49: 281-6.

[20] Hartman DS, Goldman SM, Friedman AC, et al. Angiomyolipoma: ultrasonic-pathologic correlation. Radiology 1981;139:451-8.

[21] Scheible W, Ellenbogen PH, Leopold GR, et al. Lipomatous tumors of the kidney and adrenal: apparent echographic specificity. Radiology 1978;129:153-6.

[22] Siegel CL, Middleton WD, Teefey SA, et al. Angiomyolipoma and renal cell carcinoma: US differentiation. Radiology 1996;198:789-93.

[23] Zebedin D, Kammerhuber F, Uggowitzer MM, et al. Criteria for ultrasound differentiation of small angiomyolipomas (< or =3 cm) and renal cell carcinomas. Rofo 1998;169:627-32.

[24] Yamashita Y, Ueno S, Makita O, et al. Hyperechoic renal tumors: anechoic rim and intratumoral cysts in US differentiation of renal cell carcinoma from angiomyolipoma. Radiology 1993;188:179-82.

[25] Jinzaki M, Tanimoto A, Narimatsu Y, et al. Angiomyolipoma: imaging findings in lesions with minimal fat. Radiology 1997;205: 497-502.

[26] Helenon O, Merran S, Paraf F, et al. Unusual fat-containing tumors of the kidney: a diagnostic dilemma. Radiographics 1997;17:129-44.

[27] Sant GR, Heaney JA, Ucci AA Jr, et al. Computed tomographic findings in renal angiomyolipoma: an histologic correlation. Urology 1984;24:293-6.

[28] Kim JK, Park SY, Shon JH, et al. Angiomyolipoma with minimal fat: differentiation from renal cell carcinoma at biphasic helical CT. Radiology 2004;230:677-84.

[29] Silbiger ML, Peterson CC Jr. Renal angiomyolipoma: its distinctive angiographic characteristics. J Urol 1971;106:363-5.

[30] Zagoria RJ, Dyer RB, Assimos DG, et al. Spontaneous perinephric hemorrhage: imaging and management. J Urol 1991;145:468-71.

[31] Yamakado K, Tanaka N, Nakagawa T, et al. Renal angiomyolipoma: relationships between tumor size, aneurysm formation, and rupture. Radiology 2002;225:78-82.

[32] Mourikis D, Chatziioannou A, Antoniou A, et al. Selective arterial embolization in the management of symptomatic renal angiomyolipomas. Eur J Radiol 1999;32:153-9.

[33] Kothary N, Soulen MC, Clark TW, et al. Renal angiomyolipoma: long-term results after arterial embolization. J Vasc Interv Radiol 2005; 16:45-50.

[34] Harrison RB, Dyer R. Benign space-occupying conditions of the kidneys. Semin Roentgenol 1987;22:275-83.

[35] Davis CJ Jr. Pathology of renal neoplasms. Semin Roentgenol 1987;22:233-40.

[36] Bennington JL. Proceedings: Cancer of the kidney-etiology, epidemiology, and pathology. Cancer 1973;32:1017-29.

[37] Bosniak MA. The small (less than or equal to 3.0 cm) renal parenchymal tumor: detection, diagnosis, and controversies. Radiology 1991; 179:307-17.

[38] Licht MR. Renal adenoma and oncocytoma. Semin Urol Oncol 1995;13:262-6.

[39] Quinn MJ, Hartman DS, Friedman AC, et al. Renal oncocytoma: new observations. Radiology 1984;153:49-53.

[40] Jasinski RW, Amendola MA, Glazer GM, et al. Computed tomography of renal oncocytomas. Comput Radiol 1985;9:307-14.

[41] Ambos MA, Bosniak MA, Valensi QJ, et al. Angiographic patterns in renal oncocytomas. Radiology 1978;129:615-22.

[42] De Carli P, Vidiri A, Lamanna L, et al. Renal oncocytoma: image diagnostics and therapeutic aspects. J Exp Clin Cancer Res 2000;19:287-90.

[43] Mead GO, Thomas LR Jr, Jackson JG. Renal oncocytoma: report of a case with bilateral multifocal oncocytomas. Clin Imaging 1990;14: 231-4.

[44] Zhang G, Monda L, Wasserman NF, et al. Bilateral renal oncocytoma: report of 2 cases and literature review. J Urol 1985;133:84-6.

[45] Kavoussi LR, Torrence RJ, Catalona WJ. Renal oncocytoma with synchronous contralateral renal cell carcinoma. J Urol 1985;134:1193-6.

[46] Nishikawa K, Fujikawa S, Soga N, et al. Renal oncocytoma with synchronous contralateral renal cell carcinoma. Hinyokika Kiyo 2002;48: 89–91.

[47] Dechet CB, Bostwick DG, Blute ML, et al. Renal oncocytoma: multifocality, bilateralism, metachronous tumor development and coexistent renal cell carcinoma. J Urol 1999;162:40–2.

[48] Rodriguez CA, Buskop A, Johnson J, et al. Renal oncocytoma: preoperative diagnosis by aspiration biopsy. Acta Cytol 1980;24:355–9.

[49] Nguyen GK, Amy RW, Tsang S. Fine needle aspiration biopsy cytology of renal oncocytoma. Acta Cytol 1985;29:33–6.

[50] Alanen KA, Tyrkko JE, Nurmi MJ. Aspiration biopsy cytology of renal oncocytoma. Acta Cytol 1985;29:859–62.

[51] Steiner M, Quinlan D, Goldman SM, et al. Leiomyoma of the kidney: presentation of 4 new cases and the role of computerized tomography. J Urol 1990;143:994–8.

[52] Kanno H, Senga Y, Kumagai H, et al. Two cases of leiomyoma of the kidney. Hinyokika Kiyo 1992;38:189–93.

[53] Protzel C, Woenckhaus C, Zimmermann U, et al. Leiomyoma of the kidney. Differential diagnostic aspects of renal cell carcinoma with increasing clinical Relevance. Urologe A 2001;40: 384–7.

[54] Yazaki T, Takahashi S, Ogawa Y, et al. Large renal hemangioma necessitating nephrectomy. Urology 1985;25:302–4.

[55] Fujii Y, Ajima J, Oka K, et al. Benign renal tumors detected among healthy adults by abdominal ultrasonography. Eur Urol 1995;27:124–7.

[56] Stanley RJ, Cubillo E, Mancilla Jimenez R, et al. Cavernous hemangioma of the kidney. Am J Roentgenol Radium Ther Nucl Med 1975;125: 682–7.

[57] Gordon R, Rosenmann E, Barzilay B, et al. Correlation of selective angiography and pathology in cavernous hemangioma of the kidney. J Urol 1976;115:608–9.

[58] Cubillo E, Hesker AE, Stanley RJ. Cavernous hemangioma of the kidney: an angiographic-pathologic correlation. J Can Assoc Radiol 1973;24:254–6.

[59] Roswell RH. Renin-secreting tumors. J Okla State Med Assoc 1990;83:57–9.

[60] Dunnick NR, Hartman DS, Ford KK, et al. The radiology of juxtaglomerular tumors. Radiology 1983;147:321–6.

[61] Haab F, Duclos JM, Guyenne T, et al. Renin secreting tumors: diagnosis, conservative surgical approach and long-term results. J Urol 1995; 153:1781–4.

[62] Niikura S, Komatsu K, Uchibayashi T, et al. Juxtaglomerular cell tumor of the kidney treated with nephron-sparing surgery. Urol Int 2000; 65:160–2.

[63] Weiss JP, Pollack HM, McCormick JF, et al. Renal hemangiopericytoma: surgical, radiological and pathological implications. J Urol 1984; 132:337–9.

[64] Matsuda S, Usui M, Sakurai H, et al. Insulin-like growth factor II-producing intra- abdominal hemangiopericytoma associated with hypoglycemia. J Gastroenterol 2001;36:851–5.

[65] Chung J, Henry RR. Mechanisms of tumor-induced hypoglycemia with intraabdominal hemangiopericytoma. J Clin Endocrinol Metab 1996;81:919–25.

[66] Motzer RJ, Bander NH, Nanus DM. Renal-cell carcinoma. N Engl J Med 1996;335:865–75.

[67] Smith SJ, Bosniak MA, Megibow AJ, et al. Renal cell carcinoma: earlier discovery and increased detection. Radiology 1989;170:699–703.

[68] Filipas D, Spix C, Schulz-Lampel D, et al. Screening for renal cell carcinoma using ultrasonography: a feasibility study. BJU Int 2003; 91(7):595–9.

[69] Tsuboi N, Horiuchi K, Kimura G, et al. Renal masses detected by general health checkup. Int J Urol 2000;7:404–8.

[70] Ishikawa I, Kovacs G. High incidence of papillary renal cell tumours in patients on chronic haemodialysis. Histopathology 1993;22:135–9.

[71] Sasagawa I, Nakada T, Kubota Y, et al. Renal cell carcinoma in dialysis patients. Urol Int 1994; 53:79–81.

[72] Choyke PL, Glenn GM, Walther MM, et al. Hereditary renal cancers. Radiology 2003;226: 33–46.

[73] Steffens MG, de Mulder PH, Mulders PF. Paraneoplastic syndromes in three patients with renal cell carcinoma. Ned Tijdschr Geneeskd 2004;148:487–92.

[74] Gold PJ, Fefer A, Thompson JA. Paraneoplastic manifestations of renal cell carcinoma. Semin Urol Oncol 1996;14:216–22.

[75] Kim HL, Belldegrun AS, Freitas DG, et al. Paraneoplastic signs and symptoms of renal cell carcinoma: implications for prognosis. J Urol 2003;170:1742–6.

[76] Gil H, de Wazieres B, Desmurs H, et al. Stauffer's syndrome disclosing kidney cancer: another cause of inflammatory syndrome with anicteric cholestasis. Rev Med Interne 1995; 16:775–7.

[77] Sarf I, el Mejjad A, Dakir M, et al. Stauffer syndrome associated with a giant renal tumor. Prog Urol 2003;13:290–2.

[78] Dourakis SP, Sinani C, Deutsch M, et al. Cholestatic jaundice as a paraneoplastic manifestation of renal cell carcinoma. Eur J Gastroenterol Hepatol 1997;9:311–4.

[79] Ritchie AW, Chisholm GD. The natural history of renal carcinoma. Semin Oncol 1983;10: 390–400.

[80] Amendola MA, Bree RL, Pollack HM, et al. Small renal cell carcinomas: resolving a diagnostic dilemma. Radiology 1988;166:637–41.

[81] Zagoria RJ, Wolfman NT, Karstaedt N, et al. CT features of renal cell carcinoma with emphasis

on relation to tumor size. Invest Radiol 1990; 25:261–6.

[82] Catalano C, Fraioli F, Laghi A, et al. High-resolution multidetector CT in the preoperative evaluation of patients with renal cell carcinoma. AJR Am J Roentgenol 2003;180:1271–7.

[83] Helenon O, Correas JM, Balleyguier C, et al. Ultrasound of renal tumors. Eur Radiol 2001;11: 1890–901.

[84] Yamashita Y, Takahashi M, Watanabe O, et al. Small renal cell carcinoma: pathologic and radiologic correlation. Radiology 1992;184: 493–8.

[85] Forman HP, Middleton WD, Melson GL, et al. Hyperechoic renal cell carcinomas: increase in detection at US. Radiology 1993;188:431–4.

[86] Coleman BG, Arger PH, Mulhern CB Jr, et al. Gray-scale sonographic spectrum of hypernephromas. Radiology 1980;137:757–65.

[87] Jinzaki M, Ohkuma K, Tanimoto A, et al. Small solid renal lesions: usefulness of power Doppler US. Radiology 1998;209:543–50.

[88] Ascenti G, Zimbaro G, Mazziotti S, et al. Usefulness of power Doppler and contrast- enhanced sonography in the differentiation of hyperechoic renal masses. Abdom Imaging 2001;26: 654–60.

[89] Hartman DS, Davis CJ Jr, Johns T, et al. Cystic renal cell carcinoma. Urology 1986;28: 145–53.

[90] Brinker DA, Amin MB, de Peralta-Venturina M, et al. Extensively necrotic cystic renal cell carcinoma: a clinicopathologic study with comparison to other cystic and necrotic renal cancers. Am J Surg Pathol 2000;24:988–95.

[91] Murad T, Komaiko W, Oyasu R, et al. Multilocular cystic renal cell carcinoma. Am J Clin Pathol 1991;95:633–7.

[92] Nassir A, Jollimore J, Gupta R, et al. Multilocular cystic renal cell carcinoma: a series of 12 cases and review of the literature. Urology 2002;60:421–7.

[93] Kim JC, Kim KH, Lee JW. CT and US findings of multilocular cystic renal cell carcinoma. Korean J Radiol 2000;1:104–9.

[94] Yamashita Y, Miyazaki T, Ishii A, et al. Multilocular cystic renal cell carcinoma presenting as a solid mass: radiologic evaluation. Abdom Imaging 1995;20:164–8.

[95] Kim AY, Kim SH, Kim YJ, et al. Contrast-enhanced power Doppler sonography for the differentiation of cystic renal lesions: preliminary study. J Ultrasound Med 1999;18:581–8.

[96] Habboub HK, Abu-Yousef MM, Williams RD, et al. Accuracy of color Doppler sonography in assessing venous thrombus extension in renal cell carcinoma. AJR Am J Roentgenol 1997;168:267–71.

[97] McGahan JP, Blake LC, deVere White R, et al. Color flow sonographic mapping of intravascular extension of malignant renal tumors. J Ultrasound Med 1993;12:403–9.

[98] Tsui KH, Shvarts O, Smith RB, et al. Prognostic indicators for renal cell carcinoma: a multivariate analysis of 643 patients using the revised 1997 TNM staging criteria. J Urol 2000;163: 1090–5.

[99] Cheville JC, Lohse CM, Zincke H, et al. Sarcomatoid renal cell carcinoma: an examination of underlying histologic subtype and an analysis of associations with patient outcome. Am J Surg Pathol 2004;28:435–41.

[100] Leder RA, Dunnick NR. Transitional cell carcinoma of the pelvicalices and ureter. AJR Am J Roentgenol 1990;155:713–22.

[101] Blacher EJ, Johnson DE, Abdul-Karim FW, et al. Squamous cell carcinoma of renal Pelvis. Urology 1985;25:124–6.

[102] Stein A, Sova Y, Lurie M, et al. Adenocarcinoma of the renal pelvis. Report of two cases, one with simultaneous transitional cell carcinoma of the bladder. Urol Int 1988;43:299–301.

[103] Sijmons RH, Kiemeney LA, Witjes JA, et al. Urinary tract cancer and hereditary nonpolyposis colorectal cancer: risks and screening options. J Urol 1998;160:466–70.

[104] Nocks BN, Heney NM, Daly JJ, et al. Transitional cell carcinoma of renal pelvis. Urology 1982;19:472–7.

[105] Yousem DM, Gatewood OM, Goldman SM, et al. Synchronous and metachronous transitional cell carcinoma of the urinary tract: prevalence, incidence, and radiographic detection. Radiology 1988;167:613–8.

[106] Wong-You-Cheong JJ, Wagner BJ, Davis CJ. Transitional cell carcinoma of the urinary tract: radiologic-pathologic correlation. Radiographics 1998;18:123–42.

[107] Baron RL, McLennan BL, Lee JKT, et al. Computed tomography of transitional cell carcinoma of the renal pelvis and ureter. Radiology 1982;144:125–30.

[108] Kawashima A, Vrtiska TJ, LeRoy AJ, et al. CT urography. Radiographics 2004;24:35–54.

[109] Joffe SA, Servaes S, Okon S, et al. Multi-detector row CT urography in the evaluation of hematuria. Radiographics 2003;23(6):1441–55.

[110] Subramanyam BR, Raghavendra BN, Madamba MR. Renal transitional cell carcinoma: sonographic and pathologic correlation. J Clin Ultrasound 1982;10:203–10.

[111] Kobayashi S, Ohmori M, Akaeda T, et al. Primary adenocarcinoma of the renal pelvis. Report of two cases and brief review of literature. Acta Pathol Jpn 1983;33:589–97.

[112] Wimbish KJ, Sanders MM, Samuels BI, et al. Squamous cell carcinoma of the renal pelvis: case report emphasizing sonographic and CT appearance. Urol Radiol 1983;5:267–9.

[113] Kenney PJ. Imaging of chronic renal infections. AJR Am J Roentgenol 1990;155:485–94.

[114] Kim J. Ultrasonographic features of focal xanthogranulomatous pyelonephritis. J Ultrasound Med 2004;23:409–16.

[115] Choyke PL, White EM, Zeman RK, et al. Renal metastases: clinicopathologic and radiologic correlation. Radiology 1987;162:359–63.

[116] Bhatt GM, Bernardino ME, Graham SD Jr. CT diagnosis of renal metastases. J Comput Assist Tomogr 1983;7:1032–4.

[117] Mitnick JS, Bosniak MA, Rothberg M, et al. Metastatic neoplasm to the kidney studied by computed tomography and sonography. J Comput Assist Tomogr 1985;9:43–9.

[118] Becker WE, Schellhammer PF. Renal metastases from carcinoma of the lung. Br J Urol 1986;58: 494–8.

[119] Volpe JP, Choyke PL. The radiologic evaluation of renal metastases. Crit Rev Diagn Imaging 1990;30:219–46.

[120] Hartman DS, Davidson AJ, Davis CJ Jr, et al. Infiltrative renal lesions: CT-sonographic-pathologic correlation. AJR Am J Roentgenol 1988; 150:1061–4.

[121] Paivanalo M, Tikkakoski T, Merikanto J, et al. Radiologic findings in renal metastases. Aktuelle Radiol 1993;3:360–5.

[122] Dalla Palma L, Pozzi Mucelli RS, Zuiani C. Ultrasonography and computerized tomography in the diagnosis of renal metastasis. Radiol Med (Torino) 1991;82:95–100.

[123] Honda H, Coffman CE, Berbaum KS, et al. CT analysis of metastatic neoplasms of the kidney. Comparison with primary renal cell carcinoma. Acta Radiol 1992;33:39–44.

[124] Pickhardt PJ, Lonergan GJ, Davis CJ Jr, et al. From the archives of the AFIP. Infiltrative renal lesions: radiologic-pathologic correlation. Armed Forces Institute of Pathology. Radiographics 2000;20:215–43.

[125] Fernandez-Acenero MJ, Galindo M, Bengoechea O, et al. Primary malignant lymphoma of the kidney: case report and literature review. Gen Diagn Pathol 1998;143:317–20.

[126] Porcaro AB, D'Amico A, Novella G, et al. Primary lymphoma of the kidney. Report of a case and update of the literature. Arch Ital Urol Androl 2002;74:44–7.

[127] Heiken JP, Gold RP, Schnur MJ, et al. Computed tomography of renal lymphoma with ultrasound correlation. J Comput Assist Tomogr 1983;7:245–50.

[128] Cohan RH, Dunnick NR, Leder RA, et al. Computed tomography of renal lymphoma. J Comput Assist Tomogr 1990;14:933–8.

[129] Ferry JA, Harris NL, Papanicolaou N, et al. Lymphoma of the kidney. A report of 11 cases. Am J Surg Pathol 1995;19:134–44.

[130] Richards MA, Mootoosamy I, Reznek RH, et al. Renal involvement in patients with non-Hodgkin's lymphoma: clinical and pathological features in 23 cases. Hematol Oncol 1990;8: 105–10.

[131] Horii SC, Bosniak MA, Megibow AJ, et al. Correlation of CT and ultrasound in the evaluation of renal lymphoma. Urol Radiol 1983;5: 69–76.

[132] Sheeran SR, Sussman SK. Renal lymphoma: spectrum of CT findings and potential mimics. AJR Am J Roentgenol 1998;171:1067–72.

RADIOLOGIC
CLINICS
OF NORTH AMERICA

Radiol Clin N Am 44 (2006) 805–835

ELSEVIER
SAUNDERS

Doppler Artifacts and Pitfalls

Deborah J. Rubens, MD*, Shweta Bhatt, MD,
Shannon Nedelka, MD, Jeanne Cullinan, MD

- Understanding the technical challenge of Doppler ultrasound or setting up your equipment to get the best images and spectral tracings
- Choosing the correct transducer frequency
  Doppler angle
  Sample volume
  Wall filters
  Doppler Gain
  Velocity scale
- Doppler artifacts
  Aliasing

Blooming artifact
Directional ambiguity
Partial volume artifact
Pseudoflow
Flash artifact
Mirror-image artifact
Edge artifact
Twinkling artifact
- Day-to day Doppler: too much flow versus too little flow
- Summary
- References

Thirty years ago, use of Doppler ultrasound (US) was limited to the vascular laboratory and was mainly used to interrogate the carotid arteries. Today, Doppler US has pervaded all of diagnostic US imaging, is the mainstay of venous diagnosis, and is used extensively throughout abdominal, pelvic, and obstetric imaging. In addition to continuous wave Doppler, pulsed wave (duplex) Doppler, color Doppler, and power Doppler are now available. Motion is imaged in high-velocity settings (ie, the aorta, carotid, and renal arteries) and in low flow states (portal vein thrombosis, calf veins, and so forth). Superficial structures (neck and arm vessels, testicular and ovarian vessels) and deep structures (hepatic and renal arteries) are imaged. To accomplish this range of diversity takes more than one knob on a machine. The image obtained, the particular organ being viewed, and the capabilities of the machine itself are governed by the intrinsic properties of US and Doppler. The physical properties of US give rise to several artifacts-some occur in gray-

scale and Doppler imaging and others are specific to Doppler, especially color or power Doppler. Knowing an artifact's typical location and appearance helps avoid misinterpretation and can actually be useful diagnostically [1]. Understanding how to generate a Doppler signal enables the examiner to better avoid day-to-day scanning pitfalls, which primarily fall into two clinical categories: too little flow or too much flow. This article addresses the machine parameters first, then the artifacts, and concludes with the operational issues (or pitfalls) as they apply to day-to-day scanning.

Understanding the technical challenge of Doppler ultrasound or setting up your equipment to get the best images and spectral tracings

The Doppler effect measures a change in the reflected sound frequency generated by motion of the source or the detector. The challenge lies in

This article was originally published in *Ultrasound Clinics* 1:1, January 2006.
Department of Imaging Sciences, University of Rochester Medical Center, 601 Elmwood Avenue, Rochester, NY 14642-8648, USA
* Corresponding author.
E-mail address: Deborah_Rubens@urmc.rochester.edu (D.J. Rubens).

doi:10.1016/j.rcl.2006.10.014

the detection of the signal and the accurate display of its direction and speed. Although the Doppler effect is commonly used to measure flowing blood, any tissue or fluid motion may generate a Doppler signal. That signal is a shift or difference in frequency between the transmitted and the received US pulse. The greatest difference or strongest signal is achieved when the motion is parallel to the US beam and no signal is generated when the motion is perpendicular to it.

Choosing the correct transducer frequency

Of all the technical parameters that can be controlled, the choice of transducer frequency is paramount because the intensity of the scattered sound varies in proportion to the fourth power of the Doppler frequency [2]. Higher frequencies are,

therefore, much more sensitive to flow but sometimes cannot penetrate deep enough without attenuation; thus, for superficial structures such as the testes, 7 to 10 MHz may be ideal, whereas for deep abdominal structures, such as the hepatic arteries or the portal vein, 3 MHz or lower may be needed. Often the choice of Doppler transducer frequency is empiric with a trial of different frequencies until the best compromise between penetration and signal strength is achieved [Fig. 1].

Doppler angle

Unlike in gray-scale US imaging whereby the best image is obtained perpendicular to the US beam, in Doppler US, the strongest signals (and best spectra) result when the motion is parallel to the beam. A Doppler angle of 90° does not display flow because no component of the frequency shift is

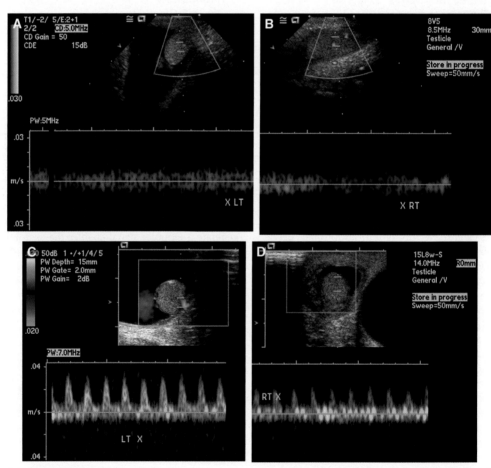

Fig. 1. Pseudotesticular torsion. Four-day-old infant presents with left hydrocele and testicular torsion is suspected. (*A*, *B*) Initial axial images of the symptomatic left (*A*) and asymptomatic right (*B*) sides at identical gain and scale settings show symmetric spectral Doppler patterns equal above and below the baseline but do not have typical vascular spectral Doppler waveform. This is noise. Note scanning frequency is 8.5 MHz and spectral Doppler frequency is 5 MHz. (*C, D*) Axial images from repeat examination with appropriate high frequency transducer shows normal symmetric arterial waveforms bilaterally. Note transducer frequency of 14 MHz and spectral Doppler frequency of 7 MHz.

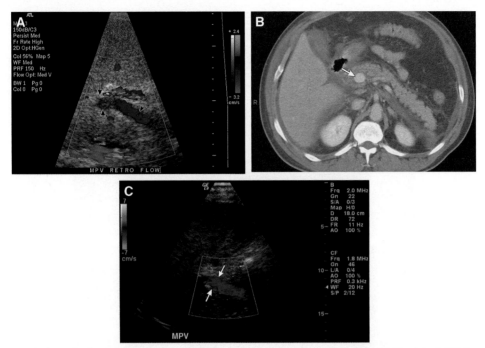

Fig. 2. Pseudothrombosis of main portal vein (MPV). (*A*) Color Doppler ultrasound (CDUS) of the MPV detects no flow in confluence of MPV (*arrows*) suggesting thrombosis of MPV. Note reversed flow in splenic vein (*arrowhead*) indicating portal hypertension and potentially slow-flow state in MPV. Wall filter set on medium, which may exclude low velocity flow and MPV segment which lacks flow is parallel to transducer surface, and therefore at 90° to Doppler beam. (*B*) Portal venous phase of subsequent contrast enhanced CT on the same day reveals completely patent MPV (*arrow*). (*C*) Repeat CDUS examination with different machine following day shows retrograde flow in MPV (*arrows*) and no apparent thrombus. Doppler angle has been improved (no longer 90°) and wall filter is corrected to low setting (20 Hz).

directed back toward the transducer [Fig. 2]. Any Doppler angle other than zero requires angle correction to adjust for the component of the signal not directed parallel to the beam. The larger the Doppler angle, the greater the correction is that needs to be done and the greater chance for error; therefore, the Doppler beam angle must always be kept as low as possible. Ideally, it should be less than 60° and always less than 70° because the errors associated with the angle correction increase up to 20% to 30% with higher Doppler angles [Fig. 3] [3].

Sample volume

The sample volume is the three-dimensional space from which the Doppler frequency shifts are measured. In color or power Doppler it is the color box, and in pulsed wave Doppler it is the cursor one places within the vessel. Although on the image the sample looks like a flat box, it has a third dimension in and out of the plane of the image, which may be much larger than anticipated (even 1 cm or more in thickness, depending on frequency and depth). Signals may be sampled and displayed from unwanted areas of a vessel (ie, too close to the vessel wall, giving more turbulence, and slower

velocities) or even from unwanted vessels (adjacent arteries or veins). In a large vessel, blood flow is not uniform across the vessel; it is generally slower near the wall (as a result of friction and turbulence) and faster in the center. Therefore, with spectral Doppler, too wide a sample (which encompasses the entire vessel lumen) includes the normal turbulence and slower velocities along the vessel margins, which result in spectral broadening (that may be incorrectly interpreted as poststenotic turbulence) [3]. If the spectral sample is too small and is not placed in the area of greatest flow, the resulting measured velocity is too low. If the sample volume is too small and the vessel is mobile, a discontinuous Doppler signal may result with loss of the diastolic signal in each cycle. The ideal sample volume size for routine survey of a vessel is about two thirds of the vessel width positioned in the center of the vessel [3] excluding as much of the unwanted clutter from near the vessel walls as possible [2].

Wall filters

The Doppler frequency shift can be detected from moving blood vessel walls and from the blood itself. These wall echoes are large amplitude causing

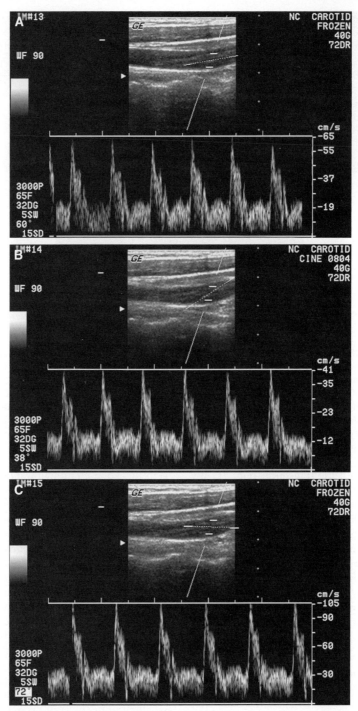

Fig. 3. Angle-corrected velocity. (*A*) Correct angle, as depicted by line through Doppler cursor, is parallel to center of lumen and yields peak systolic velocity of 65 cm/s. (*B*) Angle is too low, at 38°, which results in calculated velocity of only 41 cm/s. (*C*) Angle is only slightly off at 72° but velocity is now calculated to be 105 cm/s. Small changes in angle greater than 60° result in much larger errors than small changes below 60°.

a loud "wall thump" on the audio Doppler output [4]. Fortunately, these signals are also low frequency. By using a threshold that cuts off these low frequency noises, a cleaner high-velocity blood-flow signal is displayed; however, if the wall filter threshold is set too high, true blood flow also is discarded from the display. Low velocity venous flow and the filter for venous Doppler should be kept at the lowest practical level, usually 50 to 100 Hz or less [Fig. 2] [2].

Doppler Gain

This setting controls the amplitude of the color display in color or power Doppler mode and the spectral display in pulse Doppler mode. For spectral Doppler, the tracing should be continuous and easy to visualize, without any low-level noise band above and below the baseline. Excess spectral gain in pulse wave Doppler produces noise that may be mistaken for flow [Fig. 1]. In arterial spectra, excess gain fills in the tracing as low velocity echoes and mimics turbulent flow [5]. For color imaging, the gain should be turned up until scattered isolated color pixels can be seen overlying the gray-scale background. Then the gain should be turned back until they disappear.

If the color gain settings are too low, flow may be present but not visualized. If the settings are too high, color or power signals may overwrite gray-scale clot. A machine setting related to gain for color and power Doppler is the color-write priority. The color-write priority determines whether a given pixel is written as a gray-scale value or as color [3]. If the gray-scale signal is above some threshold (eg, medium gray), the pixel remains gray, and if the signal is below the threshold (ie, the pixel is dark gray or black), the pixel is written as color. If the gray-scale gain is too high or the color-write priority too low, some color pixels may not be displayed.

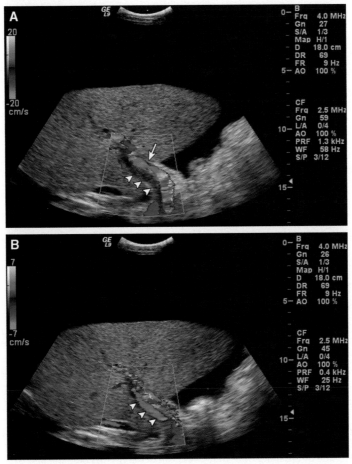

Fig. 4. Portal vein pseudoclot. (A) Longitudinal CDUS image in cirrhotic patient with portal hypertension. Velocity scale is set at 20 cm/s. Good flow in hepatic artery anteriorly (*arrow*) but none in adjacent portal vein (*arrowheads*). (B) Scale is appropriately lowered to 7 cm/s and slower flow in portal vein (*arrowheads*) can now be demonstrated.

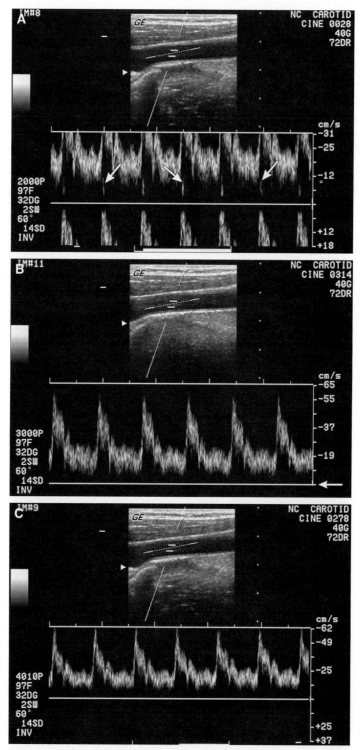

Fig. 5. Spectral aliasing. (*A*) Longitudinal spectral Doppler evaluation of common carotid artery (CCA) demonstrates spectral aliasing as higher Doppler shift frequencies "wrap around" scale and peaks (*arrows*) are written coming from opposite side of baseline. Note that peaks can actually cross baseline and overwrite existing spectral display. (*B*) Dropping baseline (*arrow*) eliminates aliasing. (*C*) Increasing scale (from 31 to 62 cm/s) eliminates aliasing.

Velocity scale

The velocity scale controls the range of frequencies displayed and is critical in color and spectral Doppler imaging. If the scale is too high (similar to a too-wide window in CT), the dynamic range is too large and low velocity signals are missed simulating an area of thrombosis [Fig. 4], particularly in low flow vessels, such as the portal vein. If the velocity scale is too low, the dynamic range is too small to display the high-velocity signals accurately and aliasing results (see later discussion).

Doppler artifacts

Doppler artifacts can be grouped into three broad categories [1]: (1) artifacts caused by technical limitations, including aliasing, improper Doppler angle with no flow, indeterminate Doppler angle, blooming, and partial volume artifact; (2) artifacts caused by patient anatomy, including mirror image artifact, flash artifact, and "pseudoflow"; and (3) artifacts caused by machine factors, including edge artifact and twinkle artifact.

Aliasing

Aliasing is an inaccurate display of color or spectral Doppler velocity and occurs when the velocity range exceeds the scale available to display it. The maximum velocity scale is limited by the number of US pulses per second that can be transmitted and received by the transducer (ie, the pulse repetition frequency [PRF]). Accurate depiction of frequency shifts requires a scale that is twice as large as the maximum shift (known as the Nyquist limit) [4]. If the scale is too small, large shifts exceed the available range and are displayed as multiples of small shifts. Practically, the display "wraps around" the scale and overwrites the existing data. For spectral Doppler flow toward the transducer, the velocity peak is cut off at the top of the scale and the

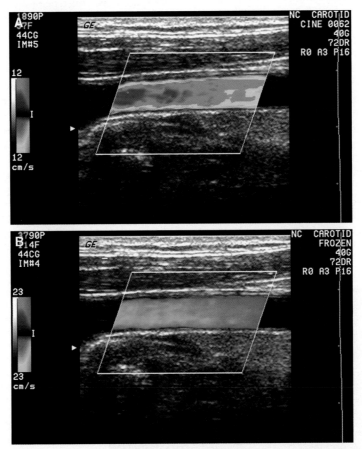

Fig. 6. Color Doppler aliasing. (*A*) Longitudinal CDUS image of CCA directed away from transducer should be red with maximum central velocity displayed as bright yellow. Instead, color scale "wraps around" and colors are displayed sequentially from red and yellow adjacent to wall to light blue and then dark blue in central lumen. Velocity scale range is 12cm/s. (*B*) At proper scale range of 23 cm/s color display no longer aliases and flow direction is depicted appropriately.

missing portion is written from the lowest portion of the scale back toward the top [Fig. 5]. The solutions to spectral aliasing are first to drop the baseline or increase the velocity scale (ie, the PRF) to increase the available velocity range [Fig. 5]. If the scale is still inadequate, decrease the Doppler frequency shift by using a lower insonating frequency or by increasing the Doppler angle [4].

For color Doppler assume a scale ranging from red (slow) to yellow (faster) toward the transducer and dark blue (slow) to light blue (faster) away. Aliasing within a vessel is displayed as adjacent colors from red to yellow to light blue to dark blue [Fig. 6]. Increasing the velocity scale [Fig. 6] or decreasing the frequency can also be diminished by color Doppler aliasing. In areas of the vessel where the flow actually reverses direction, the color palette also goes from red to dark blue but without the yellow and light blue components in between. Instead there is the black line of no flow dividing the areas in which the flow has changed direction [Fig. 7]. Power Doppler has no aliasing because it has no directional or velocity component.

Aliasing is disadvantageous in that high velocities may not be accurately measured; however, in day-to-day scanning, color Doppler aliasing can be useful because it quickly localizes the highest velocity region within a vessel for spectral sampling for carotid and other vascular studies [Fig. 8] [6]. Aliasing rapidly identifies the abnormal area in assessment of transjugular intrahepatic portal-systemic shunt TIPS [Fig. 9] and displays the direction of high-velocity jets for angle-corrected velocity determination. In addition, color Doppler aliasing readily identifies abnormal high-velocity vessels, which are often invisible on gray-scale. In particular, arteriovenous fistulae, a common sequelae to renal or hepatic biopsy [Fig. 10] [7] are often undetectable on gray-scale.

Blooming artifact

In common terms this is known as "color bleed" because the color spreads out from within the vessel and "bleeds" beyond the wall into adjacent areas. Color bleed can occur because the color US image is actually two images superimposed, the color and the gray-scale; thus, depending on how the parameters are set, the color portion of the image can extend beyond the true gray-scale vessel margin. This extension usually occurs deep to the vessels and, most commonly, is caused by abnormally high gain settings [Fig. 11] [8]. The unwanted result, however, is that the information within the vessel (ie, partial thrombus) can be "written over" and obscured. Color blooming artifact can also be seen with US contrast agents and occurs soon after the bolus injection, at the time the increase in signal strength is the highest [9]. B-flow, an alternative US-based blood flow detection method, does not use Doppler and is acquired as part of the gray-scale image; thus, the "flow" cannot overwrite the gray-scale anatomy. This type of imaging may be useful when color imaging is problematic [10].

Directional ambiguity

Directional ambiguity or indeterminate flow direction refers to a spectral Doppler tracing in which the waveform is displayed with nearly equal amplitude above and below the baseline in a mirror image pattern. This pattern results when the interrogating beam intercepts the vessel at a 90° angle [5] and is most common in small vessels, especially those that may be traveling in and out of the imaging plane [Fig. 12]. In a study by Ratanakorn and colleagues [11], this artifact adversely effected measured transcranial Doppler blood-flow velocities.

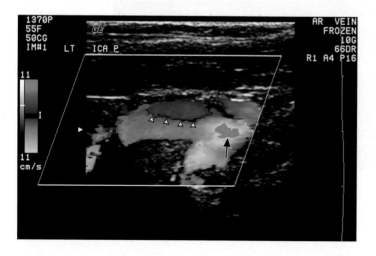

Fig. 7. Color Doppler aliasing and flow reversal. Longitudinal CDUS image of left CCA bifurcation demonstrates focal aliasing centrally (*arrow*). True flow reversal (*arrowheads*) in ICA bulb is recognized by thin black line that separates blue reversed flow near wall from adjacent red forward flow in central lumen. (*From* Zynda-Weiss A, Carson NL. Carotid arterial and vertebral Doppler ultrasound. In: Dogra V, Rubens DJ, editors. Ultrasound secrets. New York: Elsevier; 2004; with permission.)

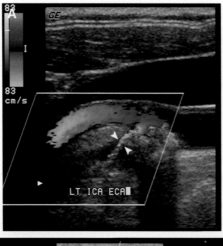

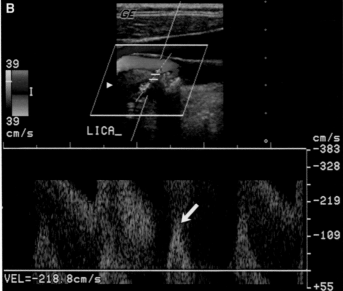

Fig. 8. Color Doppler aliasing. (*A*) Longitudinal CDUS image of left common carotid artery bifurcation demonstrates focal aliasing within ICA (*arrowheads*) indicating high-velocity jet caused by stenosis. (*B*) Spectral Doppler obtained at this region also demonstrates aliasing, even with maximized scale settings. Despite this, if peak (*arrow*) is added to portion written above baseline, velocity can be calculated at 275 + 219 = 494 cm/s, which indicates a severe stenosis. (*From* Zynda-Weiss A, Carson NL. Carotid arterial and vertebral Doppler ultrasound. In: Dogra V, Rubens DJ, editors. Ultrasound secrets. New York: Elsevier; 2004; with permission.)

Directional ambiguity should not be confused with true bidirectional flow. In the latter case, blood actually flows in two directions, such as in the neck of a pseudo-aneurysm [Fig. 13]. The clue here is that the flow is first in one direction, then in the opposite, all within a single cardiac cycle. Another type of bidirectional flow occurs in the setting of high resistance organ flow (eg, torsion, venous thrombosis, or other causes of parenchymal edema) and is represented as diastolic flow reversal [Fig. 14] [12]. The difference between true bidirectional flow and an indeterminate direction spectral tracing is that bidirectional flow is never simultaneously symmetric above and below the baseline. The flow direction varies within the cardiac cycle. True bidirectional flow is not an artifact. In the visceral arteries it is always abnormal and must be recognized to make the correct diagnosis.

Partial volume artifact

Partial volume artifact results from a slice thickness that is not infinitely thin. Echoes and Doppler signals can be acquired from objects that may be partly

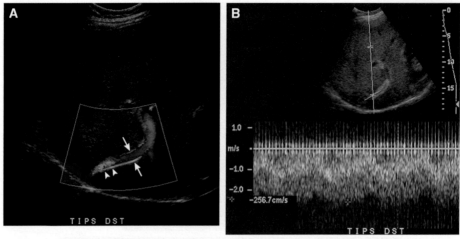

Fig. 9. Color Doppler aliasing in transjugular intrahepatic portal-systemic shunt (TIPS). (*A*) Longitudinal CDUS image of TIPS (*arrows*) demonstrates aliasing (*arrowheads*) in hepatic end of shunt suggesting focally elevated velocity. (*B*) Corresponding Doppler spectrum confirms shunt stenosis with angle- corrected flow velocity measuring 256.7 cm/s (normal velocity is <200 cm/s). (*From* Zynda-Weiss A, Carson NL. Carotid arterial and vertebral Doppler ultrasound. In: Dogra V, Rubens DJ, editors. Ultrasound secrets. New York: Elsevier; 2004; with permission.)

within the slice and partly outside of it, similar to slicing partly through a cherry in a piece of fruit cake. If viewed from one side, the slice seems to have a cherry. If viewed from the other side, no cherry seems visible. Because the signals in the US slice are summed together, the echoes produced are attributed to structures in the assumed "thin" scan plane [13]; thus, echoes can appear within anechoic structures and Doppler signals are acquired in an area in which no vessels are perceived on gray-scale [3]. For example, on a longitudinal gray-scale image, echoes from gas in the duodenum may appear within the gallbladder and mimic stones or polyps; however, if you rotate the transducer and image from the transverse plane, the gas is clearly adjacent to the gallbladder and not within it. On color flow imaging, an example of partial volume artifact is visualization of a portion of the iliac artery within the ovary giving the impression of abnormal cyst wall flow. Spectral analysis of this vessel shows the high resistance waveform typical of an iliac artery [Fig. 15] and imaging from the 90° plane clearly shows the vessel separate from the ovary. Partial volume artifact may be produced by grating lobes or side lobes, which generate information outside the expected path of the main beam. These off-axis lobes are located peripheral to the main beam axis [Fig. 16] [14]. Side lobes occur close to the primary beam whereas grating lobes can be far removed from the central beam [15]. These off-axis lobes can interrogate vessels that are separate from the primary sample volume. The lobes may appear on the spectral tracing as a flowing

vessel where none is expected or display bidirectional flow as a result of interrogating the vessel from multiple angles [Fig. 12]. These transducer related artifacts are seen mainly with the high frequency, tightly curved, convex, linear arrays used in endocavitary probes, and depend on the crystal element size and the spacing of the array elements [5].

Pseudoflow

Pseudoflow is defined as presence of flow of a fluid other than blood [7]. Pseudoflow can mimic real blood flow with color or power Doppler US, but no true vessel containing the fluid exists [Fig. 17]. The color or power Doppler signal appears as long as the fluid motion continues. These artifacts may be misinterpreted as flow unless Doppler spectral analysis is used. The spectral Doppler tracing does not exhibit a normal arterial or venous waveform [1]. Spontaneous examples of pseudoflow include ascites [Fig. 18], amniotic fluid, and urine (bladder jets). Bladder jets identify the ureteral orifice and are useful to exclude complete obstruction or to denote asymmetric ureteral emptying in the case of partial obstruction [Fig. 19] [16]. Bladder jets are not completely reliable, however, because 30% of obstructed patients may display normal jets [17]. Conversely, normal patients in the 2nd and 3rd trimester of pregnancy may have asymmetric or absent jets partly caused by uterine pressure. These jets can mostly be restored by scanning in the decubitus position, however, because the asymmetry may be physiologic and not necessarily abnormal, using

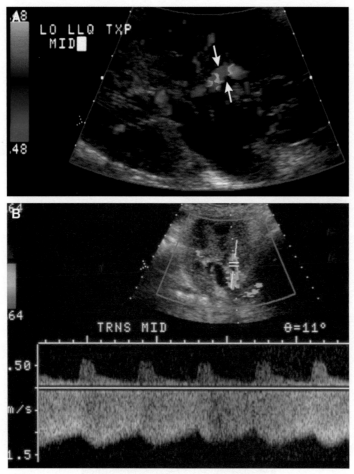

Fig. 10. Aliasing identifies an arteriovenous fistula (AVF). (*A*) Longitudinal CDUS image detects area of focal aliasing (*arrows*) indicating high-velocity flow in renal hilum, and suggests arteriovenous fistula. (*B*) Doppler spectrum demonstrates low resistance arterial waveform directed above baseline and high-velocity arterialized venous waveform below baseline, diagnostic of AVF.

diminished jets to diagnose obstruction in pregnancy still remains problematic [18].

Flash artifact

Flash artifact is a sudden burst of random color that fills the frame, obscuring the gray-scale image. This artifact may be caused by object motion or transducer motion [Figs. 20 and 21] [7]. Flash artifact may occur anywhere but is most commonly seen in the left lobe of the liver (as a result of cardiac pulsation) and in hypoechoic areas, such as cysts or fluid collections [Fig. 22] [5]. Flash artifact can be used to denote the fluid nature of solid-appearing material [Fig. 23] [1]. Power Doppler is more susceptible to flash artifact than color flow Doppler because of the longer time required to build the image (in general, more frames are averaged to create the image than with standard color Doppler) [19].

Although generally disruptive, motion artifacts can be extremely useful diagnostically. The so-called "perivascular artifact" or "color bruit" is a tissue motion artifact whereby the motion is generated within an organ, rather than involving an entire organ or image. This artifact appears as a random color mosaic in the soft tissues (as opposed to a single homogeneous color), occurs adjacent to vessels with turbulent flow, and is believed to be caused by actual vascular tissue vibration [20]. This artifact is the imaging equivalent to an auditory bruit or palpable thrill; varies with the cardiac cycle; is most prominent in systole; is absent or less prominent in diastole; is seen particularly in association with anastomotic sites, stenotic arteries, or arteriovenous fistulae [Fig. 24]; and can be extremely useful to detect their presence.

Mirror-image artifact

The mirror image artifact displays objects on both sides of a strong reflector, though they are located only on one side of it [21,22]. The reflector (eg,

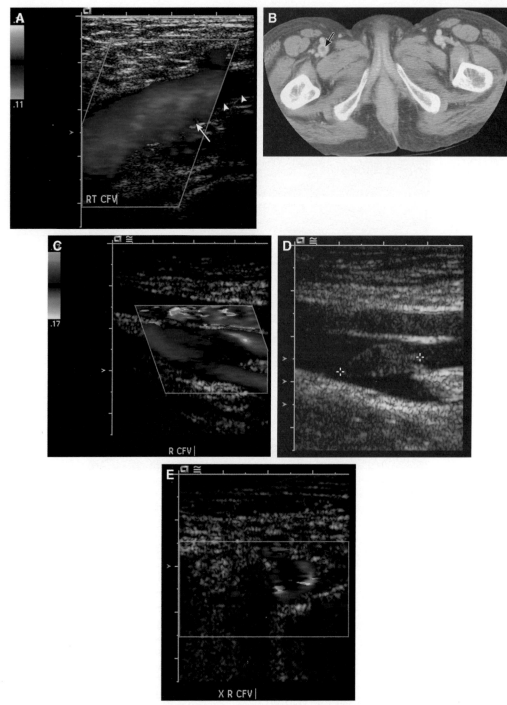

Fig. 11. Blooming artifact (*A*) Longitudinal CDUS image of right common femoral vein (CFV) shows blooming artifact deep to vessel, displaying color (*arrow*) beyond vessel wall (*arrowheads*). Color is uniform and no clot displayed. Initial examination was interpreted as normal. Scale is low at 0.11 and gain high at 50. (*B*) Axial CT just above bifurcation shows intraluminal partial thrombus (*arrow*) in right CFV. CT was obtained same day as "(*A*)". (*C*) Following CT, directed CFV CDUS was performed. Increasing scale to 0.17 and decreasing gain to 38 shows thrombus (*arrow*), which was initially missed. (*D*) Corresponding gray-scale image to C shows thrombus (*cursors*), which is larger than in CDUS image, indicating some color pixels are still overwriting gray-scale, particularly in darker portions of clot. (*E*) Axial CDUS displays thrombus centrally within CFV, identical to CT.

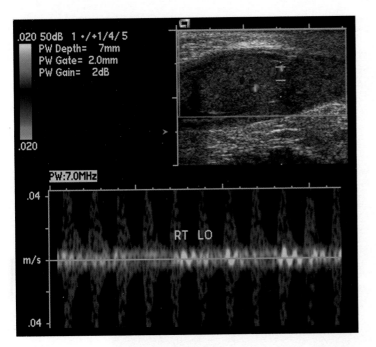

Fig. 12. Longitudinal CDUS image through infant testis shows arterial spectral Doppler waveform with equal amplitude above and below baseline, yielding an indeterminate flow direction. This occurs most often in small vessels.

the diaphragm, pleural surface, or aortic wall) directs some of the echoes to a second reflector before it returns them to the transducer, resulting in a multipath reflection [Fig. 25] [14]. The machine "straightens out" the multipath echoes assuming that the echoes come from the initial transducer beam and from a distance corresponding to the actual time of flight, resulting in a display of the echoes deeper in the image than they should be. The resulting artifact shows up as the virtual object, deep to the original image but identical to it-thus the term "mirror."

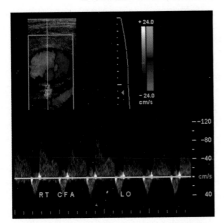

Fig. 13. True bidirectional flow in a pseudoaneurysm. Doppler spectrum at neck of pseudoaneurysm demonstrates true bidirectional flow with sequential flow first into and then out of aneurysm in each cardiac cycle.

Mirror images may be produced with gray-scale, color, power, and spectral Doppler. With Doppler, mirror image artifact commonly occurs adjacent to the highly reflective lung in the supraclavicular region [23]. Reflection off the pleura causes an apparent duplication of the subclavian artery or vein. The sound is bounced back from the surface of the lung to the moving blood cells and the resulting Doppler shift is reflected back to the surface of the lung and then to the transducer. The extra time taken causes the appearance of a second vessel deep to the real subclavian vessel, referred to as the mirror image artifact. The phantom vessel is always projected deeper in the image [Fig. 26] [5]. A carotid ghost is the term for a mirror image of the common carotid artery. The carotid ghost is always located deep to the common carotid artery regardless of location and positioning of the transducer [23].

Edge artifact

Edge artifact refers to the Doppler signal generated at the margin of a strong, smooth, specular reflector, displayed on imaging as persistent color along the rim of calcified structures, such as gallstones [Fig. 27] or cortical bone, and may mimic vascularity unless the spectral tracing is obtained [24]. Edge artifact may be generated by any echogenic surface, including manmade structures (eg, catheters and foley balloons [Fig. 28]). The diagnostic feature is the Doppler spectrum, a straight-line pattern, equal above and below the baseline, and representing noise, not flow. Edge artifact is seen more

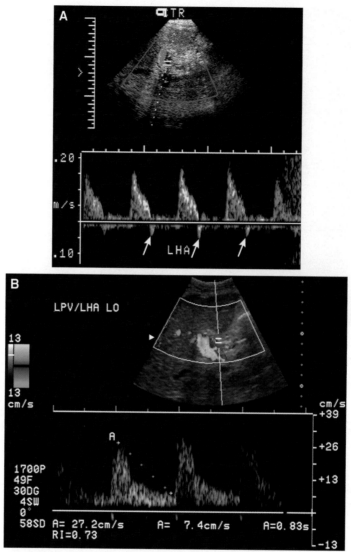

Fig. 14. Diastolic flow reversal (*A*) Spectral tracing in left hepatic artery 2 days after liver transplantation shows diastolic flow reversal (*arrows*) indicating high resistance to arterial flow. Resistive index (RI) is 1.0 (*B*) 1 day later normal continuous forward diastolic flow has been re-established and RI is normal at 0.7.

commonly with power Doppler US than with color Doppler US because of a larger dynamic range [25]. These artifacts are more frequent at low PRF or velocity scale as a result of the increased sensitivity of the system but may also be caused by a low wall filter setting [26].

Twinkling artifact

In 1996, "twinkling artifact" was described by Rahmouni and colleagues [25] as color Doppler signals that imitate motion or flow behind a stationary strongly reflecting interface. The twinkling artifact can be seen behind any granular (irregular or rough) reflecting surface but is commonly caused by renal calculi, bladder calcification, and

cholesterol crystals in the gallbladder [Fig. 29]. The twinkling Doppler is a mosaic of rapidly changing colors located deep to an echogenic reflector. With power Doppler, the signal location is the same, but the color is uniform [Fig. 30].

Twinkling artifact is believed to be caused by a narrow band of intrinsic machine noise called phase (or clock) jitter [27]. On a flat surface, system noise generates a narrow band of Doppler shift as a result of tiny clock errors. This tiny shift is usually excluded by the wall filter and, therefore, is not displayed as color. Rough surfaces increase the delays in measuring signal and amplify the errors, increasing the spectral bandwidth of this noise above the level of the wall filter. The spectrum is typical of

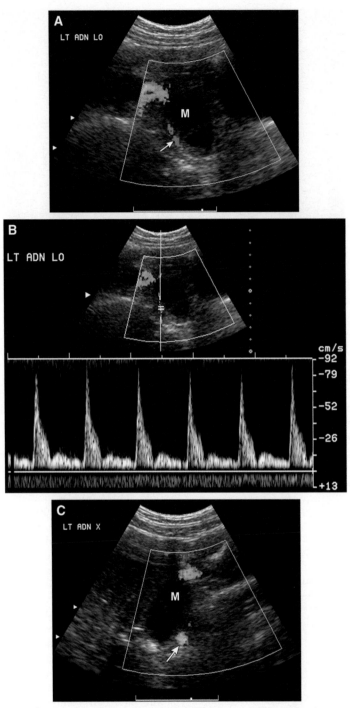

Fig. 15. Partial volume artifact in ovary. (*A*) Longitudinal CDUS image of left adnexa demonstrates vessel (*arrow*) along margin of ovarian cystic mass (M), creating concern that mass is vascular. (*B*) Doppler spectrum of this vessel reveals high resistance arterial waveform. (*C*) Axial image shows vessel (*arrows*) is actually adjacent to ovary and separate from it, not within cyst wall. (*D*) Doppler spectral waveform is identical to that in B, and is typical of internal iliac artery.

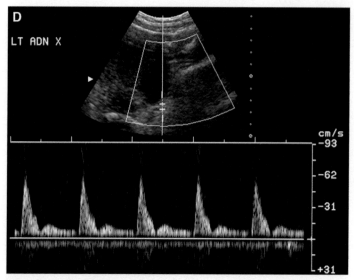

Fig. 15. (continued).

noise, with multiple closely applied spikes that are written equally above and below the baseline [Fig. 30].

Detection of the twinkling signal depends on the color-write priority and, in some instances, on gray-scale gain. As color-write priority decreases, more gray-scale is displayed, and the amount of twinkling artifact decreases behind the stone [27]. At high color-write priorities, the gray-scale has less effect. These settings vary from machine to machine and the relationships

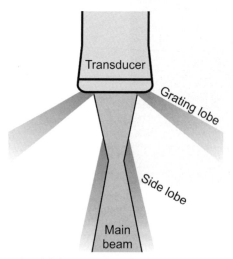

Fig. 16. Sidelobes. Diagram displays origins of side lobes and grating lobes and their relationship to main beam. Echoes returning from either of these additional lobe sources is displayed as though they originated from main beam.

between the settings also vary with manufacturer. To consistently obtain a twinkling artifact, a high color-write priority should be selected and gray-scale gain kept to a minimum.

Why produce an artifact? Unlike many artifacts that are problematic, the twinkling artifact can be extremely useful. Similar to gray-scale shadowing, twinkling artifact also may be useful to identify stones. Small stones that may not generate a strong echo or cast an acoustic shadow still can produce a twinkling artifact, leading to their identification [Fig. 31] [1]. Similar to an acoustic shadow, twinkling does not occur 100% of the time. In a study of 32 patients by Lee and colleagues [28], only 86% of urinary calculi demonstrated a twinkling artifact; furthermore, the chemical composition of stones is related to the production of the artifact. Chelfouh and colleagues [29] reported that calcium oxalate dihydrate and calcium phosphate calculi always produced a twinkling artifact, whereas stones composed of calcium oxalate monohydrate and urate lacked a twinkling artifact. Besides renal calculi, a twinkling artifact may be seen behind material with an irregularly reflective, granular surface, such as iron filings, emery paper, ground chalk, wire mesh, an aneurysm coil during transcranial Doppler sonography [30], gall bladder adenomyomatosis [31], or, recently, encrusted stents [32]. Although the twinkling artifact cannot be generated 100% of the time, it can be extremely useful in the detection of renal calculi and some foreign bodies. The key to the twinkling artifact is that the color produced *behind* the calcification and the concomitant Doppler spectral tracing shows noise, not flow; thus, a calcified carotid plaque with twinkling can

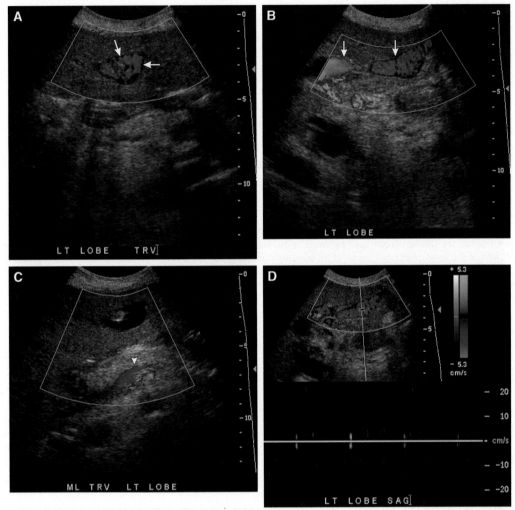

Fig. 17. Pseudoflow caused by fluid in ligamentum teres. (*A*) Transverse CDUS color flow image of liver demonstrates simulated vessel (*arrows*) coursing along falciform ligament. (*B*) Longitudinal CDUS image of same simulated vessel. (*C*) Axial image at another time point shows flow in posteriorly located splenic vein (*arrowhead*) but no flow around falciform. (*D*) Spectral Doppler tracing displays noise and no true flow. (*From* Campbell SC, Cullinan JA, Rubens DJ. Slow flow or no flow? Color and power Doppler US pitfalls in the abdomen and pelvis. Radiographics 2004;24:497-506; with permission.)

be differentiated from a potentially ulcerated plaque with flow in the ulcer cavities [Fig. 32].

Day-to day Doppler: too much flow versus too little flow

The artifacts described in the section "Doppler Artifacts" primarily relate to the generation of Doppler signals by nonvascular structures or fluids. The key to their recognition is (1) knowing that they can occur, (2) knowing the common locations and causes for their generation, and (3) identification of the nonvascular Doppler spectrum they generate, which clinches the diagnosis. In day-to-day clinical practice, the more common problems are too much

flow, which may obscure thrombi, or too little flow, giving the false diagnosis of thrombosis.

Too much flow usually can be recognized by seeing color bleed [Fig. 11], or seeing aliasing in a vessel that normally does not have it [Fig. 33]. This problem can be corrected by increasing the scale or decreasing the gain. Another common imaging problem occurs when uninterrupted flow is imaged from a segment of a vessel and flow is assumed the same throughout the rest of the lumen. This problem usually occurrs in longitudinal vascular imaging whereby a partial thrombus or atheromatous plaque may not be imaged if it is not centered in the imaging plane [Fig. 34]. The fail-safe if inappropriate settings are not recognized is always to *image in two planes;*

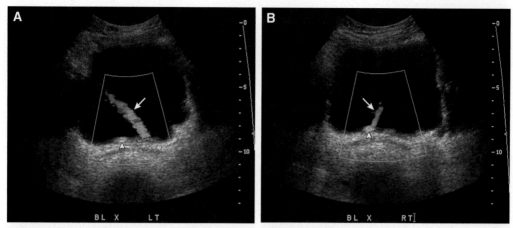

Fig. 18. Bladder jet. (*A*) Patient who presents with right renal colic. Transverse CDUS image through bladder shows normal jet (*arrow*) from asymptomatic side. Note right ureteral calculus (*arrowhead*). (*B*) Transverse CDUS image shows smaller right ureteral jet (*arrow*) indicating partial, but not complete, obstruction secondary to ureteral calculus (*arrowhead*). (*From* Campbell SC, Cullinan JA, Rubens DJ. Slow flow or no flow? Color and power Doppler US pitfalls in the abdomen and pelvis. Radiographics 2004;24:497-506; with permission.)

thus, even if the color-write priority is too high or the imaging plane is not centered and the thrombus is overwritten in the long axis of the vessel, the clot can be recognized in the short axis plane [Fig. 34].

The more common problem is too little flow, which mimics thrombosis. First, Doppler angle should be as small as possible. Obtaining signals for flow at 90° to the probe is always difficult [Fig. 2]. The scale should be set appropriately for the vessel you being interrogated. Too high a scale eliminates slow flow within the vessels [Fig. 35]. The frequency should be appropriate: low frequency for deep structures [Fig. 36] and high frequency for superficial ones [Fig. 1]. The frequency to demonstrate color flow Doppler is generally lower than the frequency needed for gray-scale imaging, so the Doppler frequency may need to be decreased if it does not default to the correct frequency. Frequency filters and other algorithms designed to decrease color tissue noise can eliminate display of slow flowing blood if they are set too high [Fig. 2]. In general, reducing the size of the color box reduces the sample size and increases the frame rate, leading to better overall sensitivity and resolution of the color image.

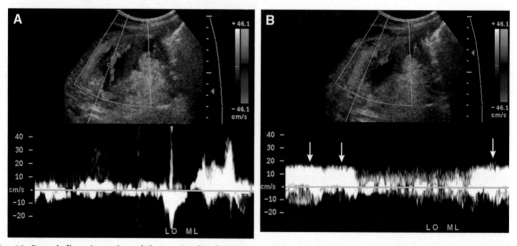

Fig. 19. Pseudoflow in ascites. (*A*) Longitudinal CDUS image in mid-abdomen in cirrhotic patient with ascites. Two linear flowing streams exist. More caudal stream (with Doppler cursor) has spectral Doppler waveform, which has random flow above and below baseline unrelated to any visceral vascular pattern. Motion in ascites occurs. (*B*) Cranial stream is continuous, unidirectional, and monophasic (*arrows*), typical of portal vein, representing patent umbilical collateral vessel. (*From* Campbell SC, Cullinan JA, Rubens DJ. Slow flow or no flow? Color and power Doppler US pitfalls in the abdomen and pelvis. Radiographics 2004;24:497-506; with permission.)

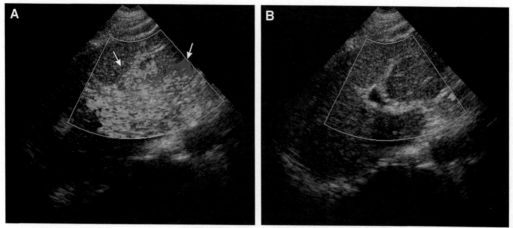

Fig. 20. Flash artifact: patient motion. (*A*) Longitudinal CDUS through the left lobe of liver with flash artifact (*arrows*) produced by respiratory motion. (*B*) Longitudinal CDUS with no motion shows normal vascular flow with no artifact.

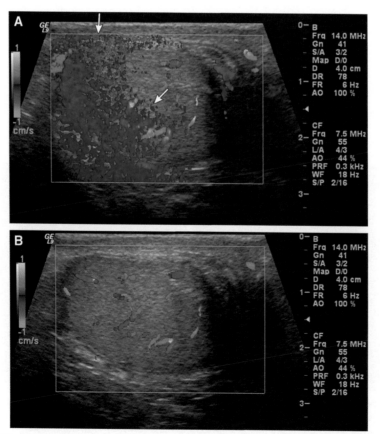

Fig. 21. Flash artifact: transducer motion. (*A*) Longitudinal CDUS of the left testis with flash artifact (*arrows*) caused by transducer motion. (*B*) Without motion, normal testicular vessels are easily identified.

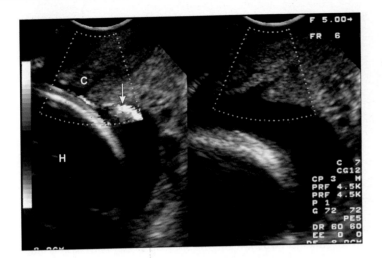

Fig. 22. Flash artifact in amniotic fluid caused by motion of fetal head. CDUS image (*left*) of lower uterine segment showing fetal head (H) and cervix (C). Flash of color (*arrow*) appears across internal os caused by application of fundal pressure while scanning, and simulates vasa previa. On corresponding CDUS image with no fundal pressure applied (*right*), no color is detected. (*From* Campbell SC, Cullinan JA, Rubens DJ. Slow flow or no flow? Color and power Doppler US pitfalls in the abdomen and pelvis. Radiographics 2004;24:497-506; with permission.)

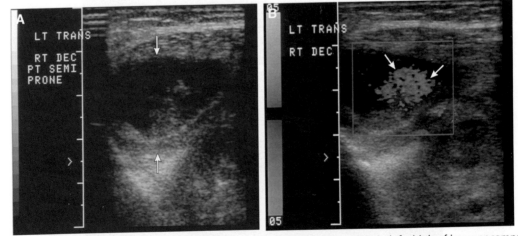

Fig. 23. Flash artifact to identify fluid for aspiration. (*A*) Transverse CDUS image in left thigh of immunocompromised patient presenting with left leg pain, originally evaluated for venous thrombosis with negative examination. Imaging in area of tenderness showed hypoechoic mass (*arrows*) with some internal echoes. (*B*) With compression applied to mass, anterior portion fills with color (*arrows*) indicating liquid, not solid mass. The apparent "mass" was aspirated and was an abscess.

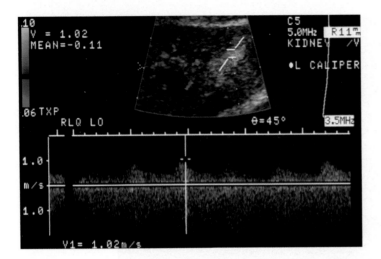

Fig. 24. Color Doppler bruit sampling in region of color Doppler bruit (mosaic of colors) shows typical spectrum of arteriovenous fistula with high-velocity arterial flow (1 m/s) and even higher venous flow (below baseline).

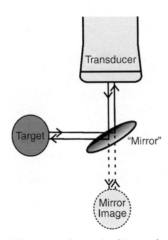

Fig. 25. Multipath reflection diagram of US wave path required to produce mirror image artifact. Pulse begins at transducer, is deflected by "mirror" (usually diaphragm or pleura) and hits target. Reflected echo returns to mirror and then to transducer, requiring much longer transit time than if pulse had interacted with object directly; thus, "mirror" image is displayed deeper in field of view.

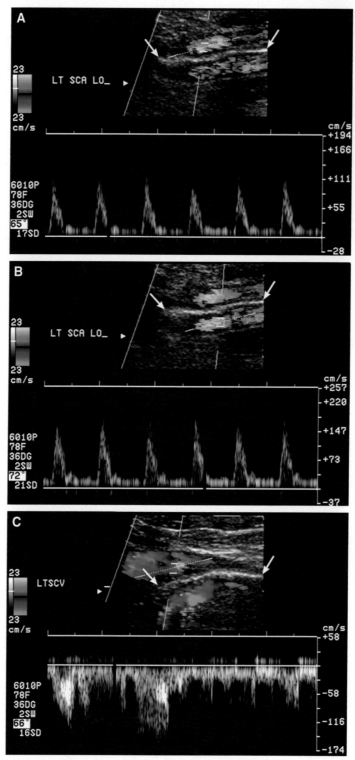

Fig. 26. Mirror-image artifact. (*A*) Anterior true vessel and (*B*) posterior mirror image of subclavian artery show identical spectra. Mirror in case is pleura (*arrows*). (*C*) Similar situation is noted with subclavian vein anteriorly and (*D*) its mirror image posteriorly with pleura (*arrows*) between them. Mirror-image vein should not be mistaken for collateral vessel.

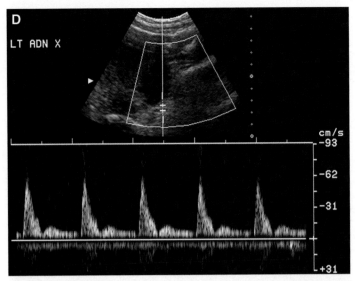

Fig. 26. (continued).

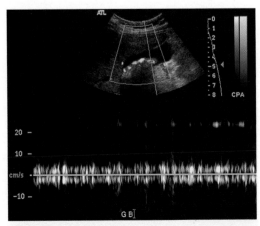

Fig. 27. Edge artifact from gallstone. Power Doppler image demonstrates color signal along rim of gallstone simulating a gallbladder mass. Spectral tracing is typical of noise, with nonvascular pattern displayed equally above and below baseline. (*From* Campbell SC, Cullinan JA, Rubens DJ. Slow flow or no flow? Color and power Doppler US pitfalls in the abdomen and pelvis. Radiographics 2004;24:497-506; with permission.)

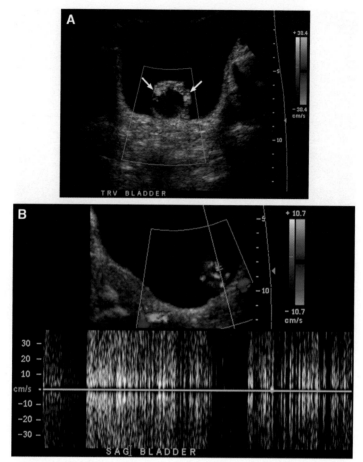

Fig. 28. Edge artifact from foley catheter. (*A*) Transverse CDUS image through bladder shows spherical mass centrally with marked Doppler signal around its margins (*arrows*). (*B*) Spectral Doppler confirms high amplitude continuous noise, equal and symmetric above and below baseline.

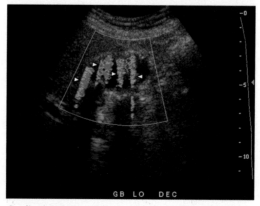

Fig. 29. Twinkling artifact longitudinal CDUS in patient with cholesterol crystals in gallbladder. Crystals generate twinkling artifact (*arrowheads*) posteriorly.

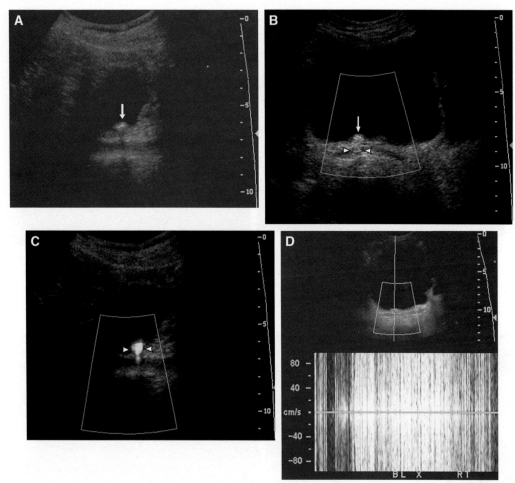

Fig. 30. Twinkling artifact. (*A*) Longitudinal image of bladder shows typical ureterovesical junction stone (*arrow*) with posterior shadow. (*B*) Transverse CDUS image of bladder shows right ureteral calculus (*arrow*) and twinkling artifact generated posteriorly (*arrowheads*). (*C*) Power Doppler also generates signal (*arrowheads*) posterior to stone. (*D*) Corresponding Doppler spectrum through twinkling color shows equal amplitude noise above and below baseline. Same spectral tracing is generated whether color or power Doppler images "twinkle." (*From* Campbell SC, Cullinan JA, Rubens DJ. Slow flow or no flow? Color and power Doppler US pitfalls in the abdomen and pelvis. Radiographics 2004;24:497-506; with permission.)

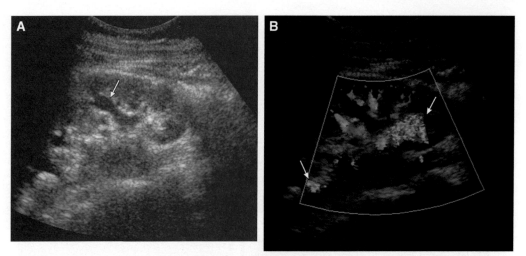

Fig. 31. Small renal stones with twinkling artifact. (*A*) Longitudinal US image through kidney shows minimal hydronephrosis (*arrow*) but no stones. (*B*) CDUS image in same position shows marked twinkling artifacts (*arrows*) at upper and lower poles, identifying stones, which do not cast an acoustic shadow.

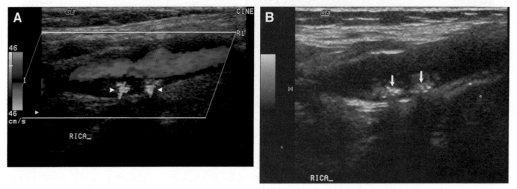

Fig. 32. Twinkling artifact in carotid. (*A*) Twinkling artifact (*arrowheads*) occurs behind calcifications (*arrows*) in atherosclerotic plaque, not to be mistaken for ulceration and disturbed flow. (*B*) Calcifications (*arrows*) are better visualized on gray-scale image. (*From* Campbell SC, Cullinan JA, Rubens DJ. Slow flow or no flow? Color and power Doppler US pitfalls in the abdomen and pelvis. Radiographics 2004;24:497-506; with permission.)

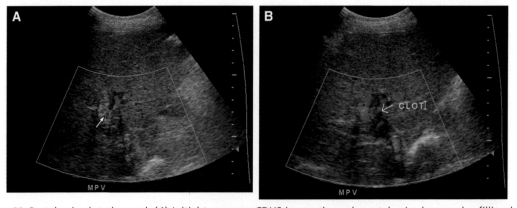

Fig. 33. Portal vein clot obscured. (*A*) Initial transverse CDUS image through portal vein shows color filling lumen; however, aliasing is occurring (*arrow*) and scale is too low at 23. (*B*) Repeat imaging with scale increased to 38 with other factors remaining constant permits detection of clot (*arrow*), which is isoechoic to liver.

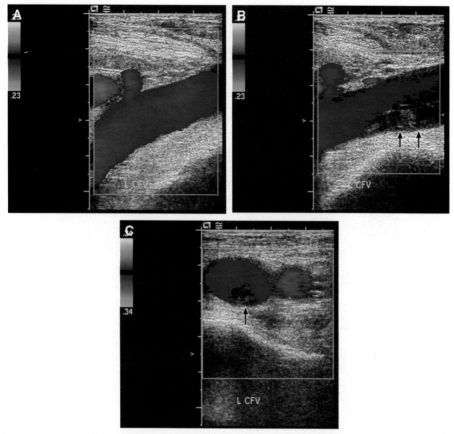

Fig. 34. Off axis imaging. (*A*) Longitudinal CDUS through common femoral vein (CFV) is normal. (*B*) With slight repositioning of transducer, large partial thrombus is identified posteriorly (*arrows*). (*C*) Transverse imaging shows partial thrombus centered in vein. Imaging in sagittal plane angled either side of thrombus creates false negative diagnosis.

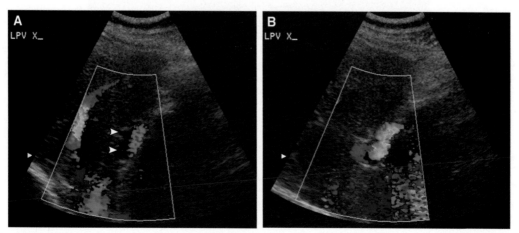

Fig. 35. Partial thrombus in left portal vein? (*A*) Initial transverse CDUS image shows only partial filling of left portal vein, simulating a thrombus (*arrowheads*) on right wall. Mean velocity scale is 17cm/s, too high for slow-flowing portal vein. (*B*) Repeat transverse image with scale at 10 cm/s shows normal filling of vein and no thrombus.

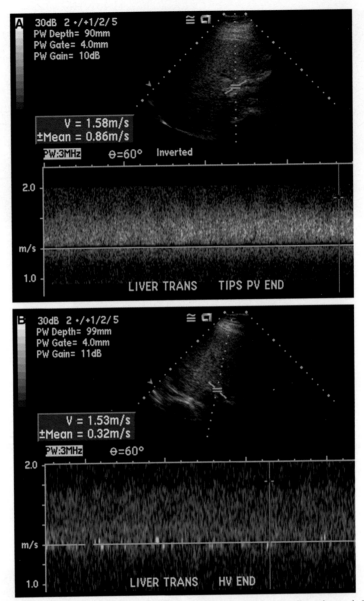

Fig. 36. No flow in central TIPS. (*A*) Initial longitudinal spectral Doppler sampling through TIPS shows normal inflow at portal vein end. (*B*) Hepatic vein portion also has normal flow. (*C*) In mid TIPS between hepatic and portal venous segments, there is no demonstrable flow. Spectral frequency is 3 MHz (*arrow*). (*D*) Normal flow in mid TIPS is documented using frequency of 2 MHz (*arrow*).

RADIOLOGIC
CLINICS
OF NORTH AMERICA

Radiol Clin N Am 44 (2006) 837–861

ELSEVIER
SAUNDERS

First-Trimester Screening

David A. Nyberg, MD[a],*, Jon Hyett, MD[b],
Jo-Ann Johnson, MD, FRCSC[c], Vivienne Souter, MD[d]

All patients have a 2% to 3% risk of birth defects, regardless of their prior history, family history, maternal age, or lifestyle [1]. Chromosome abnormalities account for approximately 10% of birth defects, but are important because of their high mortality and morbidity. Trisomy 21 (Down syndrome) is the most common serious chromosome abnormality at birth, occurring in approximately 1 of 500 pregnancies in the United States. The actual risk varies with maternal and gestational age and whether there is a history of previous pregnancies affected by chromosomal abnormality, although, as with other birth defects, all patients are at risk for fetal Down syndrome.

A detailed fetal anatomic survey performed at 18 to 22 weeks remains the primary means for detecting the majority of serious "structural" birth defects; however, first-trimester screening at 11 to 14 weeks has developed into the initial screening test for many patients. A wealth of information can be obtained at this time, including detection of many structural defects, as well as screening for fetal aneuploidy, including Down syndrome. The major advantage of first-trimester screening is the earlier gestational age of detection so that diagnostic testing (chorionic villous sampling [CVS] or genetic amniocentesis) can be made available for patients considered at highest risk for chromosome abnormalities. First-trimester screening can also help identify patients at increased risk for a variety of other abnormalities, including cardiac defects, that may be seen later. In this way, first-trimester screening can help triage patients for subsequent testing.

Older screening methods relied on clinical risk factors, particularly maternal age, to determine which patients might benefit from a diagnostic invasive test for fetal aneuploidy; however, maternal age alone is a poor screening method for determining who is at risk for chromosome abnormalities.

This article was originally published in *Ultrasound Clinics* 1:2, April 2006.
[a] Fetal and Women's Center of Arizona, 9440 E. Ironwood Square Drive, Scottsdale, AZ 85258, USA
[b] Maternity Services, Royal Brisbane Women's Hospital, Butterfield Street, Herston GLD 4006, Australia
[c] Department of Obstetrics and Gynecology, Calgary, AB, Canada
[d] Good Samaritan Medical Center, 1111 East McDowell Road, Phoeniz, AZ 85006, USA
* Corresponding author.
E-mail address: nyberg@u.washington.edu (D.A. Nyberg).

doi:10.1016/j.rcl.2006.10.017

First-trimester screening has proved to be very effective in screening for fetal aneuploidy. The accuracy of both first-trimester and second-trimester ultrasound can be improved by also considering various biochemical markers. As a result, there are currently four main components to screening for fetal aneuploidy and other birth defects: (1) first-trimester ultrasound, (2) first-trimester biochemistry, (3) second-trimester ultrasound, and (4) second-trimester biochemistry. These four components of contemporary screening can be used in isolation or can be combined with one another for greater accuracy.

This article focuses on first-trimester ultrasound screening, but also describes related screening protocols that can be used.

First-trimester aneuploidy screening

It is now well-known that increased fluid or thickening beneath the skin at the back of the neck is associated with a higher risk for fetal aneuploidy and other birth defects. This sonographic observation mirrors the clinical description of Down syndrome made more than 100 years ago by Dr. Langdon Down, who reported that the skin of affected individuals is "too large for their bodies" [2].

During the 1980s, many ultrasound studies described the typical appearance of cystic hygromas in the second trimester, and their association with aneuploidy, particularly Turner's syndrome [2–12]. At the same time, it was observed that cystic hygromas seen during the first trimester may have different appearances (nonseptated), and different associations (trisomies) than those seen during the second trimester. It was also observed that "cystic hygromas" seen during the first trimester can resolve to nuchal thickening alone, or even normal nuchal thickness, and still be associated with aneuploidy [13,14]. In a related observation, Benacerraf and colleagues [15,16] noted that second-trimester nuchal thickening was associated with an increased risk of Down syndrome.

In 1992, Nicolaides and colleagues [17] proposed the term "nuchal translucency (NT)" for the sonographic appearance of fluid under the skin at the back of the fetal neck observed in all fetuses during the first trimester [Fig. 1]. They further reported an association between the thickness of the translucency and the risk of fetal aneuploidy, especially trisomies. This concept of measuring NT in all fetuses formed the basis for first-trimester screening by ultrasound. By 1995, the first large study of NT was published [18]. Subsequent studies have confirmed that NT thickness can be reliably measured at 11 to 14 weeks gestation and, combined with maternal age, can produce an effective means of screening for trisomy 21 [19].

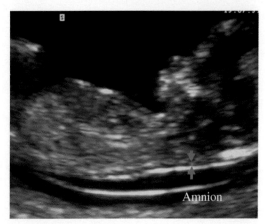

Fig. 1. Normal nuchal translucency measurement (*arrows*) at 12 weeks, 5 days.

The mechanism for increased NT may vary with the underlying condition. The most likely causes include heart strain or failure [20,21] and abnormalities of lymphatic drainage [22]. Evidence for heart strain includes the finding of increased levels of atrial and brain natriuretic peptide mRNA in fetal hearts among trisomic fetuses [23]. Also, some Doppler ultrasound studies of the ductus venosus at 11 to 14 weeks in fetuses who have increased NT have reported absent or reversed flow during atrial contraction in the majority of chromosomally abnormal fetuses and in chromosomally normal fetuses who have cardiac defects [24,25].

Abnormal lymphatic drainage may occur because of developmental delay in the connection with the venous system, or a primary abnormal dilatation or proliferation of the lymphatic channels. Fetuses who have Turner's syndrome are known to have hypoplasia of lymphatic vessels [26,27]. Lymphatic drainage could also be impaired by lack of fetal movements in various neuromuscular disorders, such as fetal akinesia deformation sequence [28].

An alternative explanation for increased NT is abnormal composition of the extracellular matrix. Many of the component proteins of the extracellular matrix are encoded on chromosomes 21, 18, or 13. Immunohistochemical studies of the skin of chromosomally abnormal fetuses have demonstrated specific alterations of the extracellular matrix that may be attributed to gene dosage effects [29,30]. Altered composition of the extracellular matrix may also be the underlying mechanism for increased fetal NT in certain genetic syndromes that are associated with alterations in collagen metabolism (such as achondrogenesis Type II), abnormalities of fibroblast growth factor receptors (such as achondroplasia and thanatophoric dysplasia), or disturbed metabolism of peroxisome biogenesis factor (such as Zellweger syndrome).

All studies indicate that proper training is required to obtain reproducible, accurate data from NT measurements [31–33]. The Fetal Medicine Foundation (www.fetalmedicine.org) has outlined guidelines that have become the standard for measurement of NT throughout the world. These are listed in Box 1. They also offer a certificate of competency for those sonographers who successfully show they can adhere to them. Virtually identical guidelines have now been proposed by the Society for Maternal Fetal Medicine in the United States, and they also offer a certificate of competency.

Use of the guidelines proposed by the Fetal Medicine Foundation have resulted in a high consistency in results [Table 1]. Monni and coworkers [34] reported that after modifying their technique of measuring NT, by following the guidelines established by The Fetal Medicine Foundation, their detection rate of trisomy 21 improved from 30% to 84%.

The ability to measure NT and obtain reproducible results improves with training; good results are achieved after 80 and 100 scans for the transabdominal and the transvaginal routes, respectively [35]. The intraobserver and interobserver differences in measurements are less than 0.5 mm in 95% of cases [36]. NT is usually measured using a transabdominal approach; transvaginal scanning may be necessary in 5% to 10% of pregnancies when transabdominal scans are technically limited.

The normal range for NT measurements is gestational age dependent. Pandya and colleagues [36] reported that the median NT increases from 1.3 mm at a crown-rump length (CRL) of 38 mm to 1.9 mm at a CRL of 84 mm. The 95th percentile increases from 2.2 mm at a crown rump length of 38 mm to 2.8 mm at a CRL of 84 mm. Sonographers should recognize that technical factors influence NT measurements. For example, extension of the neck increases NT thickness, whereas flexion reduces the measurement.

The criteria for a positive NT scan have evolved since its first description. Initially a categorical cut-off measurement (usually 2.5 or 3 mm) was used by most centers; however, as noted above, NT increases with gestational age, and the degree of risk was found to vary with NT measurements. Therefore, it is more appropriate to express NT measurements relative to gestational age or CRL as a delta value or multiple of the median. Use of multiple of median data and derived likelihood ratios can then estimate the patient-specific risk. This also permits integration of risk based on NT with biochemical data to generate a combined risk. It should be noted that the median NT measurement for Down syndrome is about two multiples of the median. This is equivalent to about 2.5 mm at 12 weeks.

The effectiveness of NT screening for detection of fetal Down syndrome has now been confirmed by a number of studies [see Table 1]. In the largest multicenter study published [19], 96,127 singleton pregnancies were examined, including 326 affected by trisomy 21 and 325 who had other chromosomal abnormalities. The median gestation at the time of screening was 12 weeks (range 10–14 weeks), and the median maternal age was 31 years (range 14–45 years). The fetal NT was above the 95th percentile for crown-rump length in 72% of the trisomy 21 pregnancies [Figs. 2, 3]. The estimated risk for trisomy 21 based on maternal age and fetal NT was above 1 in 300 in 8.3% of normal pregnancies and 82% of those affected by trisomy 21. For a screen positive rate of 5%, the sensitivity was 77% (95% CI: 72%–82%). The cumulative data from a number of other studies demonstrate a sensitivity of 77% for a false positive rate of 3% [see Table 1] [37–46].

The effectiveness of screening for fetal aneuploidy is further increased when nuchal translucency thickness is combined with biochemical markers [Table 2]. The two most effective maternal serum markers currently used in the first trimester are pregnancy-associated plasma protein A (PAPP-A) and free B-human chorionic gonadotrophin (B-hCG). Maternal serum free β-human chorionic gonadotropin (β-hCG) normally decreases with gestation after 10 weeks and maternal serum PAPP-A levels normally increase. Levels of these two proteins tend to be increased and decreased, respectively, in pregnancies affected by trisomy 21. There does not appear to any correlation between the rise in free β-hCG and fall in PAPP-A seen in trisomy 21 pregnancies, so these markers may be combined for screening purposes [47]. Similarly, these biochemical markers are independent of fetal NT thickness, allowing combination of biochemical and ultrasound tests [48,49].

Box 1: **Criteria for what constitutes an adequate NT measurement include**

1. Crown-rump length between 45 mm and 84 mm
2. Sagittal view that shows the nuchal measurement and face with the fetus in neutral position
3. Magnification so that only the upper two thirds of the fetus is included on the image
4. Distinguishing nuchal membrane from the amnion
5. Measuring maximal subcutaneous translucency overlying the neck
6. Identifying causes of falsely increased nuchal translucency measurements, including fetal extension, and nuchal cord

Table 1: **Studies examining the implementation of fetal nuchal translucency measurement at 10–14 weeks of gestation in screening for trisomy 21**

Author	N	Screening cutoff	FPR	DR
Pandya et al, 1995 [37]	1763	NT >2.5 mm	3.6%	3 of 4 (75%)
Szabo et al, 1995 [38]	3380	NT >3.0 mm	1.6%	28 of 31 (90%)
Taiplae et al, 1997 [39]	6939	NT >3.0 mm	0.8%	4 of 6 (67%)
Hafner et al, 1998 [40]	4233	NT >2.5 mm	1.7%	3 of 7 (43%)
Pajkrt et al, 1998 [41]	1473	NT >3.0 mm	2.2%	6 of 9 (67%)
Economides et al, 1998 [42]	2281	NT >99th centile	0.4%	6 of 8 (75%)
Zoppi et al, 2000 [43]	5210	Risk >1 in 100	4.2%	33 of 47 (70%)
Thilaganathan et al, 1999 [44]	11,398	Risk >1 in 200	4.7%	16 of 21 (76%)
Schwarzler et al, 1999 [45]	4523	Risk >1 in 270	4.7%	10 of 12 (83%)
Theodoropoulos et al, 1998 [46]	3550	Risk >1 in 300	4.9%	10 of 11 (91%)
Total	44,750		3.0%	119 of 156 (76%)

Abbreviations: DR, detection rate; FPR, false-positive rate; N, number.

Some authorities believe it is important to distinguish cystic hygromas from increased NT [50], whereas others do not. Malone and coworkers [50] reported 132 cases of cystic hygroma with follow-up among 38,167 screened patients (1 in 289). Chromosomal abnormalities were diagnosed in 67 (51%), including 25 who had Down syndrome, 19 who had Turner's syndrome, 13 who had trisomy 18, and 10 who had other types of chromosome abnormalities. Major structural fetal malformations, primarily cardiac and skeletal abnormalities, were diagnosed in 22 of the remaining 65 cases (34%). Of the remaining cases, 20 resulted in spontaneous fetal death (n = 5) or elective pregnancy termination (15). One of 23 normal survivors (4%) was diagnosed with cerebral palsy and developmental delay at birth. Overall, survival with normal pediatric outcome was confirmed in 17% of cases (22 of 132). Compared with increased nuchal translucency (>3

mm), cystic hygromas carried a fivefold, 12 fold, and sixfold increased risk of aneuploidy, cardiac malformation, and perinatal death, respectively. On the other hand, cystic hygromas were associated with larger NT measurements than those that had increased NT but did not have cystic hygromas, so it remains uncertain whether cystic hygromas are an independent risk factor. Like patients who have increased NT, the vast majority of pregnancies that have normal evaluation at the completion of the second trimester resulted in a healthy infant and a normal pediatric outcome.

Lateral neck cysts, also termed "jugular lymphatic sacs," have been found by Bekker and coworkers [51] to be associated with larger NT measurements and thus a higher risk for fetal aneuploidy [Fig. 4]. They found that among 26 fetuses with increased NT (> 95th percentile), 22 had clearly visible jugular lymphatic sacs and 16 of 26 (62%) had aneuploidy.

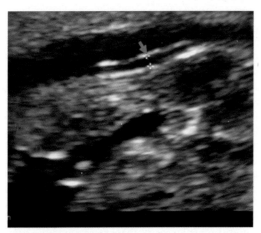

Fig. 2. Mildly increased nuchal translucency measurement associated with trisomy 21 (*calibers*). The nuchal measurement was 2.3 mm, which is about twice normal for gestational age. Biochemical values also indicated an increased risk for trisomy 21.

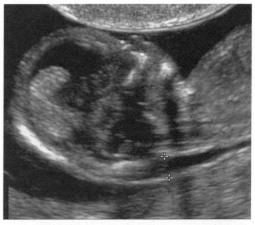

Fig. 3. Increased nuchal translucency and trisomy 21. The nuchal translucency measurement (*NT*) exceeded 3 mm.

Table 2: **Studies examining the implementation of a combined first-trimester test using maternal age, fetal nuchal translucency thickness, free β-hCG and PAPP-A to screen for trisomy 21**

Author	N	FPR	DR
Orlandi et al, 1997 [53]	744	5.0%	6 of 7 (86%)
Biagotti et al, 1998 [54]	232	5.0%	24 of 32 (75%)
Benattar et al, 1999 [55]	1656	5.0%	5 of 5 (100%)
De Biasio et al, 1999 [56]	1467	3.3%	11 of 13 (85%)
De Graff et al, 1999 [57]	300	5.0%	31 of 37 (84%)
Spencer et al, 1999 [47]	1156	5.0%	187 of 210 (89%)
Krantz et al, 2000 [58]	5718	5.0%	30 of 33 (90%)
Total	11,273	4.8%	294 of 337 (87%)

In comparison, two fetuses in the control group also showed jugular lymphatic sacs and their NT measurements were upper normal (2.8 mm and 2.9 mm). Although one might conclude that lateral neck cysts are associated with a high risk of fetal aneuploidy, Sharony and colleagues [52] found that the outcome of lateral neck cysts is associated with both the presence of other abnormalities and the NT measurement, but not with the presence of cysts themselves. On the other hand, these authors found a relatively high incidence of lateral neck cysts (2.4%) in the general population, suggesting that some of these cysts were very small and would have escaped general detection.

Screening strategies

First-trimester combined screen

The first-trimester combined screen uses maternal age, NT measurement, and biochemical markers

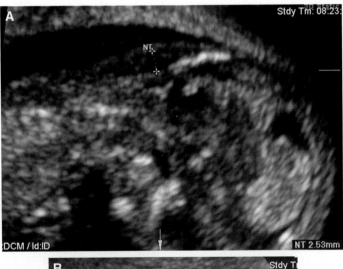

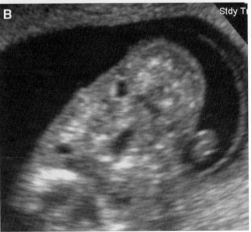

Fig. 4. Distended jugular lymphatic "sacs." (*A*) Increased nuchal translucency measurement of 2.5 mm is noted. (*B*) Transvaginal scans show small bilateral fluid collections consistent with jugular lymphatic sacs. These are associated with increased nuchal translucency measurements.

(free β-hCG and PAPP-A) to estimate the risk for fetal Down syndrome and trisomy 18. This is the most popular and effective screening strategy during the first trimester. A number of studies suggest a detection rate in the range of 85% to 90% for a screen positive rate of 5% [see Table 1] [52–59].

Two large US studies have also been reported showing the effectiveness of first-trimester screening. The First-trimester Maternal Serum Biochemistry and Fetal Nuchal Translucency Screening (BUN) study found a 79% detection rate, for a 5% false-positive rate [60].

The First- and Second-Trimester Evaluation of Risk (FASTER) Research Consortium trial [61] is the largest US-based study, and the only study that has compared first-trimester screening with second-trimester screening. The FASTER data [61] clearly confirm the pioneering work of Nicolaides and colleagues [17,19], with similar results. The overall detection rate was 85%, for a false-positive rate of 5%; however, the results clearly varied with gestational age, with detection rate of 87% at 11 weeks compared with 82% at 13 weeks.

First-trimester combined screen plus other ultrasound markers

Although increased NT remains the primary ultrasound marker of fetal aneuploidy and other birth defects during the first trimester, several other ultrasound findings have been found to be helpful at this time. These include hypoplastic or absent nasal bone, and abnormal Doppler waveforms of the tricuspid valve and ductus venosus.

Hypoplastic/absent nasal bone

A small nasal bone was first noted to a common feature of patients who had trisomy 21 by Dr. Langdon Down [2]. Anthromorphic studies in patients who have trisomy 21 have shown a small nasal bone in approximately half of affected cases. A number of ultrasound studies have now also shown an association between sonographically absent nasal bone and trisomy 21 as well as other chromosome abnormalities [62–69]. In the combined data of 15,822 fetuses, the fetal profile was successfully examined in 97.4%, and the nasal bone was absent in 1.4% of normal fetuses and in 69% of fetuses who had trisomy 21.

A minority of studies have concluded that an absent nasal bone is not a useful feature to detect fetal Down syndrome, and that reproducibility is poor during the first trimester [70,71]. This probably reflects the technical difficulty in obtaining accurate nasal bone measurements at this time. Imaging of the nasal bones requires a near-perfect midsagittal image and optimal angle of insonation with the fetal profile, whereas NT measurements can be obtained with minor variations off-center and differences in direction of imaging. Demonstrating the absence of a very small structure is even more difficult than detecting its presence, because it can be difficult to know for certain whether the nasal bones are absent or whether the images are simply suboptimal. Malone and coworkers [71] found that factors associated with an increased failure rate of nasal bone included early gestational age when the nasal bone is normally small, larger maternal body habitus, inadequate nuchal translucency sonography, and use of a transvaginal sonographic approach.

Increased impedance of flow of the ductus venosus

Abnormal Doppler flow patterns of the ductus venosus have been associated with an increased risk of fetal Down syndrome [Fig. 5] [24,25]. Matias and colleagues [24] performed ductus venosus Doppler measurements on 486 singleton fetuses, including 68 who had chromosomal abnormalities, at 10 to 14 weeks' gestation. In 90.5% of the chromosomally abnormal fetuses there was reversed or absent flow during atrial contraction, whereas abnormal ductus flow was only present in 3.1% of the chromosomally normal fetuses. The height of the A-wave was found to be the only significant independent factor in multivariate regression analysis. Other researchers have also found that ductus venosus Doppler studies can substantially improve Down syndrome screening efficiency [72].

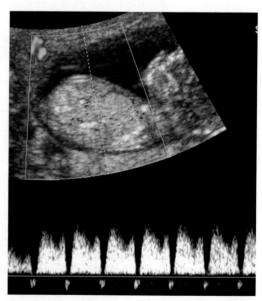

Fig. 5. Abnormal ductus venosus Doppler and trisomy 21 (same fetus as Fig. 4). Duplex Doppler of the ductus venosus shows retrograde flow during atrial contractions.

Tricuspid regurgitation has also been associated with an increased risk of fetal Down syndrome. In the largest study reported, Faiola and coworkers [73] reported that the tricuspid valve was successfully examined in 718 (96.8%) cases. Tricuspid regurgitation was found in 39 (8.5%) of the 458 chromosomally normal fetuses, in 82 (65.1%) of the 126 who had trisomy 21, in 44 (53%) of the 83 who had trisomy 18 or 13, and in 11 (21.6%) of the 51 who had other chromosomal defects. In chromosomally normal fetuses, tricuspid regurgitation was associated with increased NT measurements, suggesting that Doppler studies may be particularly useful in this group of patients.

Fetuses who have abnormal flow patterns of the ductus venosus and tricuspid valve also appear to have a higher risk of cardiac defects. Among 142 chromosomally normal fetuses who had increased NT, 11 fetuses had reversed or absent flow on ductus venosus Doppler during atrial contraction, and 7 of these had major cardiac defects at subsequent echocardiography [25]. Similarly, Faiola and colleagues [73] found that in the chromosomally normal fetuses, tricuspid regurgitation was found in nearly half (46.9%) of fetuses who had cardiac defects and in 5.6% of those who did not have cardiac defects (likelihood ratio of 8.4).

Nicolaides and coworkers [74] suggest that secondary findings of absent nasal bone or abnormal Doppler studies could be particularly useful in patients found to be in the intermediate risk group by the first-trimester screen. Using these secondary signs in patients with an intermediate risk group (risk of 1 in 100 to 1 in 1000) for fetal Down syndrome, the researchers reported detection rates of 92% for absent nasal bone, 94% for increased impedance of the ductus venosus, and 91.7% for tricuspid regurgitation, with each method showing an overall false-positive rate of less than 3% [74].

First-trimester screening followed by second-trimester biochemistry

Second-trimester biochemical screening can detect 70% to 80% of affected fetuses who had Down syndrome (at a false positive rate of 7%–8%). The effectiveness appears to be clearly higher for the "quad" screen (HCG, alpha-fetoprotein, estriol, and inhibit-A), than the older "triple" screen that did not include inhibin-A [50]; however, the effectiveness of second-trimester biochemical screening is more limited in a population that has already been screened, and in the authors' experience, most patients who have undergone first-trimester screening will choose not to undergo second-trimester biochemical screening.

For those patients who would like additional reassurance by way of a second-trimester biochemical screen, it should be done in a way that accounts for the first-trimester screening results rather than treating them as independent tests. One method is the so-called "integrated screen," which combines the elements of the first-trimester combined screen with the elements of the second-trimester "quad" screen, providing a single, low false-positive result in the second trimester [75]. This is the most accurate screening method currently available, with detection rate of 92% in the FASTER study [76]; however, a major disadvantage of integrated screening is that patients do not receive results until after completion of the second-trimester biochemistry. Thus screen-positive women do not have the option of CVS for early definitive diagnosis [77]. In addition, it is considered unethical to suppress ultrasound information obtained in the first trimester.

"Stepwise sequential" screening is an alternative approach that has been proposed; it interprets second-trimester results based on first-trimester risk assessment. A clear advantage of stepwise sequential screening is that it provides some women an earlier diagnosis while maintaining an extremely high detection rate. This method has gained rapid acceptance and it is expected to be widely adapted into clinical practice in the near future [78]. When patients in the FASTER trial underwent first-trimester combined screening at 11 weeks and the false-positive rate of each component was set at 2.5%, stepwise sequential screening provided a 95% detection of Down syndrome, for a 4.9% false-positive rate. This compares to a 4.0% false-positive rate for fully integrated screening.

Incorporation of second-trimester biochemical as part of a stepwise sequential screen would be most effective for patients considered in an intermediate risk group (risk between 1 in 100 and 1 in 1000) [79]. The intermediate group includes 15% of affected fetuses who had Down syndrome and approximately 15% of normal fetuses. In comparison, high risk patients (risk > 1 in 100) should probably consider diagnostic invasive testing without additional screening; this group includes 80% of affected fetuses who have Down syndrome but only 5% of normal fetuses. Also, low-risk patients (risk < 1 in 1000) probably do not require additional screening in most cases; this group of patients includes less than 5% of affected fetuses who have Down syndrome, but 80% of normal fetuses.

First-trimester screening followed by second-trimester ultrasonography

A second-trimester fetal survey remains the primary method of detecting the majority of birth defects that can be detected prenatally [80]. Because of the wide range of anomalies that can be detected at this time, this examination is unlikely to be replaced by any other screening test in the future. In addition to detection of structural defects, the presence or absence of various sonographic markers can further modify the risk for fetal aneuploidy, including Down syndrome. The estimated risk can be derived by multiplying the background risk (based on maternal age, gestational age, history of previously affected pregnancies, and, where appropriate, the results of previous screening by NT or biochemistry in the current pregnancy) by the likelihood ratio of the specific defect [81]. The most common second-trimester ultrasound markers that are systematically evaluated include nuchal thickening, echogenic intracardiac foci, absent or hypoplastic nasal bone, hyperechoic bowel, renal pyelectasis, and shortened femur and humerus lengths relative to the biparietal diameter. Nyberg and coworkers [82] and others have calculated likelihood ratios for many of these markers and have refined this for single markers [83].

In the vast majority of cases, second-trimester ultrasound markers such as echogenic intracardiac foci will be found in normal fetuses, especially when the marker is isolated. In this situation, a prior normal first-trimester screening result can be very reassuring. Because a normal first-trimester screening results permits significant reduction of risk for fetal Down syndrome, and because isolated findings such as echogenic intracardiac foci only slightly increase the risk, most patients will remain at very low risk and do not require further testing. Ultrasound findings, however, can also improve the detection rate of fetuses who have Down syndrome in patients who have borderline normal results from first-trimester screening, or fetuses who show multiple markers or major defects. At the same time, a normal second-trimester ultrasound can reduce the risk of fetal Down syndrome

approximately threefold, and this can normalize patients who have borderline positive results form first-trimester screening (risk 1 in 100 to 1 in 300).

Results of the FASTER trial show that use of a second-trimester genetic sonogram can both improve the detection rate and lower the false positive rate in patients who have undergone first-trimester screening [84].

Other advantages of first-trimester screening

Other chromosome abnormalities

Nuchal translucency is also increased with other chromosome abnormalities, including trisomies 13 and 18, Turner's syndrome, triploidy, and unbalanced translocations [Fig. 6] [85]; however, first-trimester biochemical markers may differ from those typically associated with trisomy 21. In trisomies 18 and 13, maternal serum free β-hCG and PAPP-A are decreased [86,87]. In cases of sex chromosomal anomalies, maternal serum free β-hCG is normal and PAPP-A is low [88]. Triploidy of paternal origin, which is associated with a partial molar placenta, has greatly increased levels of free β-hCG, whereas PAPP-A is mildly decreased [89]. In contrast, digynic triploidy, characterized by severe asymmetrical fetal growth restriction, is associated with markedly decreased maternal serum free β-hCG and PAPP-A. Screening by a combination of fetal NT, free β-hCG, and PAPP-A can identify about 90% of these anomalies for a screen positive rate of 1%.

Birth defects in euploid fetuses who have increased nuchal translucency

Extensive studies have now established that, in chromosomally normal fetuses, increased NT is

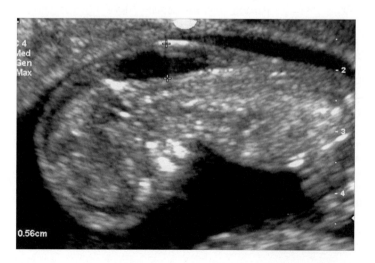

Fig. 6. Increased nuchal translucency and trisomy 18. Large nuchal translucency measurement was noted and cytogenetic testing revealed trisomy 18.

0.56cm

Table 3: Abnormalities and genetic syndromes reported in association with increased nuchal translucency and normal karyotype

Central nervous sytem defect	Anencephaly
	Craniosynostosis
	Dandy-Walker malformation
	Diastematomyelia
	Encephalocele
	Holoprosencephaly
	Hydrolethalus syndrome
	Joubert syndrome
	Microcephaly
	Macrocephaly
	Spina bifida
	Iniencephaly
	Trigoncephaly C
	Ventriculomegaly
Facial defect	Agnathia/micrognathia
	Facial cleft
	Treacher-Collins syndrome
Nuchal defect	Cystic hygroma
	Neck lipoma
Cardiac defect	Di George syndrome
Pulmonary defect	Cystic adenomatoid malformation
	Diaphragmatic hernia
	Fryn syndrome
Abdominal wall defect	Cloacal exstrophy
	Omphalocele
	Gastroschisis
Gastrointestinal defect	Crohn's disease
	Duodenal atresia
	Esophageal atresia
	Small bowel obstruction
Genitourinary defect	Ambiguous genitalia
	Congenital nephrotic syndrome
	Hydronephrosis
	Hypospadius
	Infantile polycystic kidney disease
	Meckel-Gruber syndrome
	Megacystis
	Multicystic dysplastic kidney disease
	Renal agenesis
Skeletal defect	Achondrogenesis
	Achondroplasia
	Asphyxiating thoracic dystrophy
	Blomstrand osteochondrodysplasia
	Campomelic dwarfism
	Jarcho-Levin syndrome
	Kyphoscoliosis
	Limb reduction defect

Table 3: (*continued*)

Central nervous sytem defect	Anencephaly
	Noonan-Sweeney syndrome
	Osteogenesis imperfecta
	Roberts syndrome
	Robinow syndrome
	Short rib polydactyly
	Sirenomelia
	Talipes equinovarus
	Split hand/foot malformation
	Thanatophoric dwarfism
	VACTER association
Fetal anemia	Blackfan-Diamond anemia
	Dyserthropoietic anemia
	Fanconi anemia
	Parovirus 19 infection
	Alpha thalassemia
Neuromuscular defect	Fetal akinesia deformation sequence
	Myotonic dystrophy
	Spina muscular atrophy
Metabolic defect	Beckwith-Wiedemann syndrome
	GM1 gangliosidosis
	Long-chain 3-hydroyacyl-coenzyme A dehydrogenase deficiency
	Mucopolysaccharisosis Type VII
	Smith-Lemli-Opitz syndrome
	Vitamin D-resistant rickets
	Zellweger syndrome
Other	Body stalk anomaly (limb body wall complex)
	Brachmann-de Lange syndrome
	CHARGE association
	Deficiency of the immune system
	Congenital lymphedema
	EEC syndrome
	Neonatal myoclonic encephalopathy
	Noonan syndrome
	Perlman syndrome
	Stickler syndrome
	Unspecified syndrome
	Severe developmental delay

Abbreviation: EEC syndrome, ectrodactyly-ectodermal dysplasia-cleft palate syndrome.
Adapted from Souka AP, Krampl E, Bakalis S, et al. Outcome of pregnancy in chromosomally normal fetuses with increased nuchal translucency in the first-trimester. Ultrasound Obstet Gynecol 2001;18(1):13, 14.

Table 4: Nuchal translucency measurements and adverse outcomes

Nuchal translucency measurement	Aneuploidy	Death	Major anomaly	Alive and well
<95th percentile	.2%	1.3%	1.6%	97%
95th–99th	3.7%	1.3%	2.5%	93%
3.5–4.4 mm	21.1%	2.7%	10%	70%
4.5–5.4 mm	33.3%	3.4%	18.5%	50%
5.5–6.4%	50.5%	10.1%	24.2%	30%
6.5 mm	64.5%	19%	46.2%	15%

Data from Refs. [19,42,90,103].

associated with a wide range of fetal defects and genetic syndromes [Table 3].

The prevalence of birth defects and adverse outcome also increases with increasing NT measurements [Table 4]. Souka and colleagues [90] reported that the overall risk of adverse outcome, including miscarriage and intrauterine death, was 32% for those who had NT of 3.5 to 4.4 mm, 49% for NT of 4.5 to 5.4 mm, 67% for NT 5.5 to 6.4 mm, and 89% for those who had NT of 6.5 mm or more. Among 1080 surviving fetuses who had NT of 3.5 mm or more, 5.6% had abnormalities requiring medical or surgical treatment or leading to mental handicap. The chance of no defect among live births was 86% for those who had NT of 3.5 to 4.4 mm, 77% for those who had NT of 4.5 to 5.4 mm, 67% for those who had NT of 5.5 to 6.4, and 31% for those who had NT of 6.5 mm or more.

An association between increased NT and cardiac defects was first noted by Hyett and coworkers [20] in both chromosomally abnormal and normal

fetuses. This has subsequently been confirmed by a number of studies [91–100]. A retrospective study of 29,154 chromosomally normal singleton pregnancies identified major defects of the heart and great arteries in 50 cases, and 56% of these had NT measurement translucency above the 95th percentile [101]. In chromosomally normal fetuses, the prevalence of major cardiac defects increases exponentially from 1.6 per 1000 for NT less than 95th percentile, 1% for NT between 2.5 and 34 mm, 3% for NT 3.5% to 4.4%, 7% for NT 4.5% to 5.4%, 20% for NT 5.5 to 6.4 mm, 30% for NT 6.5 mm or more.

The clinical implication of these observations is that patients found to have increased NT should undergo formal fetal echocardiography. Certainly, the overall prevalence of major cardiac defects in such a group of fetuses (about 2%) is similar to that found in pregnancies affected by maternal diabetes mellitus or who have a history of a previously affected offspring, which are well-accepted indications for fetal echocardiography. Improvements in

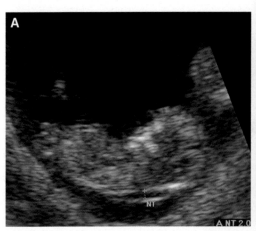
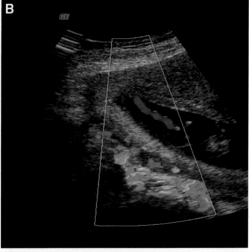

Fig. 7. Discrepant nuchal translucency measurements in monochorionic twins. (*A*) This fetus shows nuchal translucency measurement (*NT*) of 2 mm at 12 weeks. The co-twin showed nuchal translucency measurement of 1.1 mm. (*B*) Velemenous cord insertion is also apparent. This monochorionic twin pregnancy showed signs of severe twin-twin transfusion syndrome by 18 weeks.

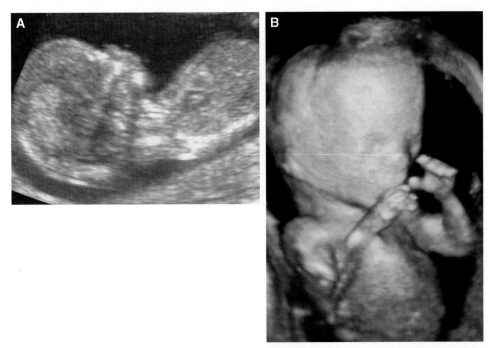

Fig. 8. Normal face at 13 weeks. (A) Sagittal view shows normal facial profile including nasal bone. (B) 3D multiplanar ultrasound with surface rendering shows normal facial features.

the resolution of ultrasound machines have now made it possible to undertake detailed cardiac scanning as early as 14 weeks [87,102].

It should be emphasized to the parents that increased NT per se does not constitute a fetal abnormality, and that, once chromosomal defects have been excluded, nearly 90% of liveborns who have fetal translucency below 4.5 mm have healthy live births. If the fetus survives until midgestation, and

if a targeted ultrasound at 20 to 22 weeks fails to reveal any abnormality, the risk of adverse outcome is not statistically increased [103]. The rate of development delay is also not statistically increased among fetuses who have increased NT [104].

Twins and multiple gestations

First-trimester screening can be effectively used for twin pregnancies [105]. Detection rates for Down

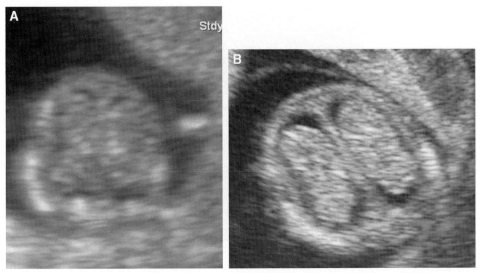

Fig. 9. Normal brain at 12 weeks. (A) Transabdominal scans show that the normal choroid plexus dominates the cerebral hemispheres. (B) Transvaginal scan on the same patient better shows normal anatomy.

syndrome are in the range of 75% to 85%, with a 5% false-positive rate [106]. Therefore, effective screening and diagnosis of major chromosomal abnormalities can be achieved in the first-trimester, allowing the possibility of earlier and therefore safer selective feticide for those parents that choose this option.

Discrepant NT measurements also appear to be a nonspecific early marker of twin-twin transfusion syndrome among monochorionc twins [Fig. 7]. In a study of 132 monochorionic twin pregnancies, including 16 that developed severe twin-to-twin transfusion syndrome at 15–22 weeks of gestation, increased NT (above the 95th percentile of the normal range) at the 11 to 14 week scan was associated with a fourfold increase in risk for the subsequent development of severe twin-to-twin transfusion syndrome [107]. It is possible that increased NT thickness in the recipient fetus may be a manifestation of heart failure caused by hypervolemic

congestion. With advancing gestation and the development of diuresis that would tend to correct the hypervolemia and reduce heart strain, both the congestive heart failure and NT resolve.

Severe complications unique to monochorionic pregnancies, such as reversed arterial perfusion syndrome or acardiac twin, and conjoined twins, can be diagnosed during the first trimester. Twin reversed arterial perfusion (TRAP) has been reported at 10 to 12 weeks using both TVS and color Doppler [108,109]. Conjoined twins have also been frequently diagnosed during the first trimester, and have been detected as early as 8 to 9 weeks [110–118].

Structural defects detected during the first trimester

Use of a systematic survey can demonstrate normal anatomic development in the first trimester, similar to the fetal survey performed during the second

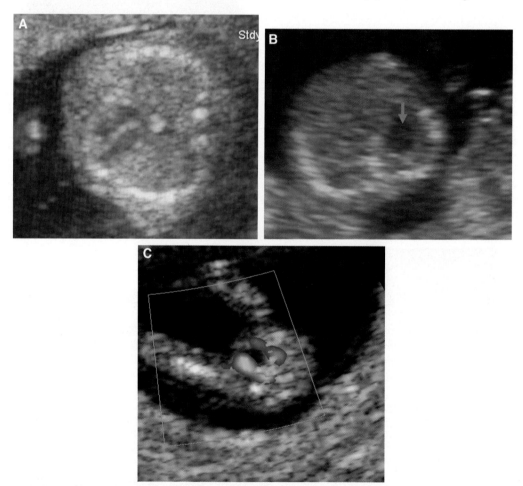

Fig. 10. Normal anatomy. (*A*) Transvaginal scan at 13 weeks shows normal four-chamber view of the heart. (*B*) Transabdominal scan at 13 weeks shows normal fluid-filled stomach. (*C*) Transabdominal scan of the pelvis at 12 weeks shows a normal urinary bladder between the two umbilical arteries, seen with color flow Doppler. A normal urinary bladder is less frequently seen than the stomach.

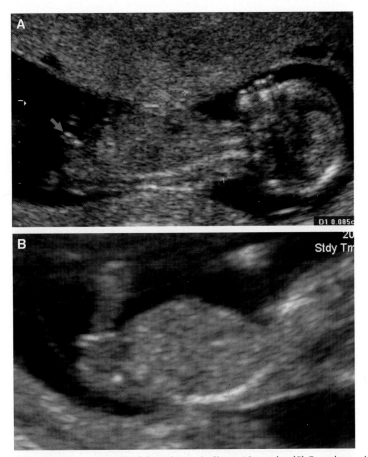

Fig. 11. Normal genitalia. (A) Male genitalia at 13 weeks. (B) Female genitalia at 12 weeks.

trimester. Normal structures that can be visualized include the brain, choroid plexi, posterior fossa, face, heart, thorax, abdomen, stomach, urinary bladder, and all four extremities, including both feet and hands [Figs. 8–10]. In addition, the individual digits of each hand can usually be counted by 12 weeks. Fetal gender can be reliably determined by 13 weeks, and by 12 weeks in most cases [Fig. 11] [119]. When deviation from normal anatomy is recognized, a number of birth defects can be detected during the first trimester. Detection varies significantly between centers, with increasing detection by a thorough systematic survey and greater use of transvaginal ultrasound and three-dimensional (3D) multiplanar ultrasound.

Ossification of the fetal cranium begins and accelerates after 9 weeks [120,121], so that anencephaly can be diagnosed as early as 9 to 10 weeks [122]. Ancephaly can also be easily overlooked during the first trimester, however, because it initially is seen as acrania with absent calvarium but relatively normal amount of brain. Careful scrutiny will show an abnormal shape and appearance of the brain caused

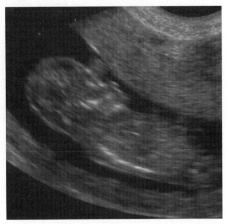

Fig. 12. Anencephaly/acrania at 12 weeks. The normal calvarium is not visualized and the shape of the brain is slightly abnormal. Anencephaly/acrania can be easily missed at this gestational age.

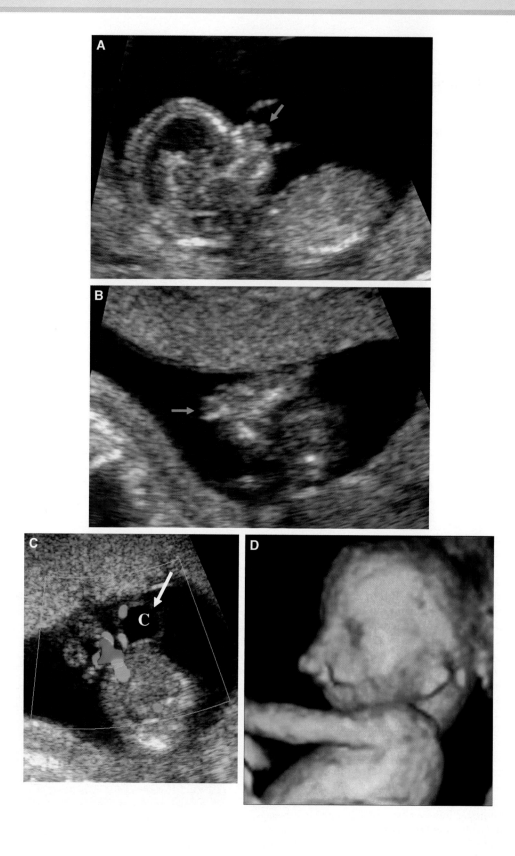

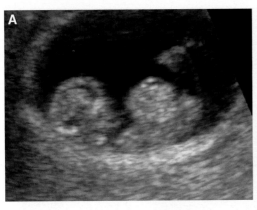

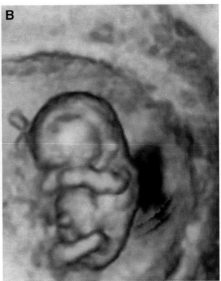

Fig. 14. (*A, B*) Omphalocele associated with trisomy 18 at 10.5 weeks. Chorionic villus sampling showed trisomy 18.

by the lack of the supporting calvarium [Fig. 12]. The sagging appearance of the brain may show "Mickey Mouse" ears.

Posterior cephaloceles have been diagnosed as early as 12 weeks [123], and alobar holoprosencephaly has been diagnosed as early as 10 weeks [124,125], but other brain abnormalities cannot reliably detected until later.

Spina bifida can occasionally be detected before the 12th postmenstrual week by noting irregularities of the bony spine or a bulging within the posterior contour of the fetal back [126]. There are also well-established additional sonographic findings that can enhance the detection of spina bifida, namely "the lemon sign" or "the banana sign" [127,128], and these may be evident as early as 12 weeks, although they can be initially subtle [129–131]. With high quality imaging, which may include tansvaginal scans, a normal posterior cerebellum and cisterna magna should be apparent, and this finding excludes all but the mildest forms of spina bifida.

Cleft lip and palate have been diagnosed in utero as early as the 13 to 14 weeks [132]. Bilateral cleft lip and palate may appear initially only as a an echogenic median mass, which actually is the pre-maxillary protrusion, made up of soft tissue, and

at times of osseous and dental structures [Fig. 13] [133]. Because bilateral cleft lip and palate is associated with a high rate of aneuploidy and other birth defects, close follow-up, genetic counseling, and amniocentesis should be offered.

Ocular abnormalities such as hyper- and hypotelorism, anophthalmia and microphthalmia, have been diagnosed from 12 to 16 weeks [134–136]. Congenital cataracts has been diagnosed as early as 12 to 14 weeks [137,138].

By 12 to 14 weeks, a four-chamber view of the heart can be consistently imaged [95,97,139,140]. The great arteries can also be imaged by 11 to 12 weeks in many cases. As with normal anatomy later in the second trimester, the right and left ventricles should be of approximately the same size, the heart should not occupy more than one third of the thoracic cavity, and the heart apex should be oriented obliquely to the left anterior thorax. Achiron and colleagues [98] reported eight cases of heart defects among approximately 1000 fetuses scanned by transvaginal ultrasound between 10 and 12 weeks. Only one fetus had an abnormal karyotype (45XO), but all fetuses showed other anomalies. Based on this experience, detection of isolated heart abnormalities is likely to remain difficult before 14 weeks.

Fig. 13. Bilateral cleft lip associated with trisomy 13 at 13 weeks. (*A*) Sagittal view shows abnormal soft tissue protruding just below the nose (*arrow*). (*B*) Transverse view confirms this finding. Bilateral cleft lip and palate was diagnosed (*arrow*). (*C*) Umbilical cord cyst (*arrow, C*) was also noted. (*D*) Follow-up 3D rendered image at 17 weeks confirms bilateral cleft lip and palate with premaxially protrusion. Other findings identified on the follow-up ultrasound, but not seen on the first-trimester scan, included echogenic intracardiac focus in the left ventricle, mildly hypoplastic left ventricle and atrium, micro-opthalmia, echogenic kidneys, and polydactyly.

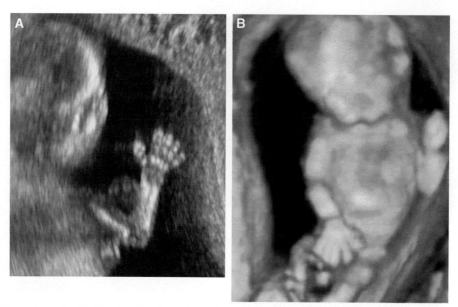

Fig. 15. Normal hands. (*A*) 2D ultrasound at 12 weeks, 3 days shows normal hand with four fingers and one thumb. (*B*) Another fetus at 13 weeks shows normal hand and extremities with 3D surface rendering.

Abdominal and truncal defects may be diagnosed during the first trimester, and these include omphalocele, gastroschisis [141,142], ectopia cordis [143,144], and body-stalk anomaly [145,146]. Omphaloceles may be categorized as those containing both bowel and liver (extracorporeal liver) and those containing only bowel (intracorporeal liver). Intracorporeal omphalocele can only be reliably diagnosed after 12 postmenstrual weeks, because of the difficulty in distinguishing it from physiologic midgut herniation [147,148]. Such omphaloceles have a high rate of fetal aneuploidy [149,150]. Extracorporeal omphalocele can be diagnosed as early as 9 to 10 weeks [151–153], and these may also be associated with fetal aneuploidy and other birth defects, including cardiac defects [Fig. 14].

The kidneys assume their final position within the renal fossa by 11 weeks [154]. Using transvaginal ultrasound, the kidneys can be consistently imaged by 12 to 13 weeks [155–157]. Cystic kidneys can sometimes be diagnosed during the first trimester. Multicystic dysplastic kidney disease has been

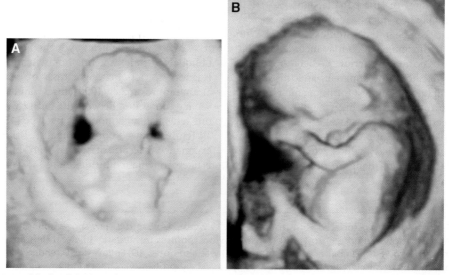

Fig. 16. Normal limbs. (*A*) 3D surface rendering image shows poor visualization of extremities. (*B*) Transvaginal scans better shows normal extremities.

diagnosed as early as 12 to 15 weeks [157]. Infantile polycystic kidney disease has also been diagnosed by 13 to 16 weeks by demonstration of enlarged, echogenic kidney. [158,159], although oligohydramnios may not develop until after 16 weeks.

The urinary bladder becomes apparent at 10 to 12 weeks, but like the kidney, it does not become consistently imaged until the 13th week [159], at which time cyclical filling and emptying of the fetal bladder should be apparent. Obstructive uropathy at the level of the urethra results in an enlarged urinary bladder (megacystis), which has been diagnosed as early as the 11th week [160,161]. It has been suggested that the diagnosis of megacystis can be reliably diagnosed when the urinary bladder measures more than 15 mm during the first trimester [162]. Affected fetuses seen during the first trimester have a high rate of associated anomalies and aneuploidy [163].

The limbs begin to develop toward the end of the sixth week with development of the upper limbs before the lower limbs [164], and they can be imaged by the eighth week [165]. By 12 weeks the hands, fingers, feet, and toes can be consistently imaged [Fig. 15]. Use of transvaginal sonography and 3D ultrasound with surface rending can aid in visualization of the extremities [Fig. 16]. By the 12th week, the long bones, phalanges, ilium, and scapula begin to ossify; the metacarpals and metatarsals ossify by 12 to 16 weeks [166]. Active fetal movements

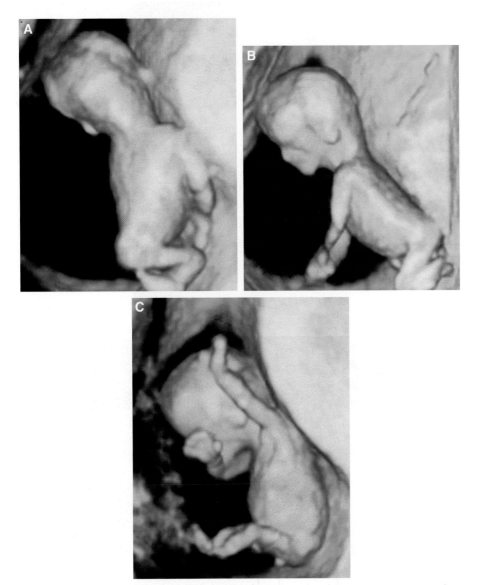

Fig. 17. Normal extremity movements at 13 weeks. Three images obtained within a few seconds of one another (*A, B, C*) show normal extremities with active normal movement.

can be observed after 10 weeks [167]. Normal fetal activity is particularly apparent using real-time 3D ("4D") ultrasound with surface rendering [Fig. 17].

A variety of skeletal abnormalities can be detected during the first trimester, including amputation defects and certain lethal skeletal dysplasias [Fig. 18]; however, their detection clearly varies with gestational age. In one of the largest reported series of prenatally diagnosed skeletal abnormalities in the first and early second trimesters, Bronshtein and co-workers [168] were able to detect 96% of the anomalies between 14 to 16 weeks, 3% between 12 to 14 weeks, and 1% at 10 to 12 weeks. Osteogenesis imperfecta (OI) is one of the lethal skeletal dysplasias

that has been diagnosed as early as 13 to 15 weeks [169–172]. Sirenomelia has been diagnosed as early as 11 to 14 weeks using transvaginal ultrasound [173–176]. It is expected that akensia can be detected during the first trimester. Polydactyly can also be detected during the first trimester, and this can be aided by use of 3D multiplanar ultrasound.

Summary

Screening for fetal chromosome abnormalities, particularly for trisomy 21, has made dramatic advances in the last 15 years. These advances have

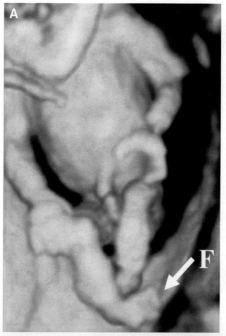

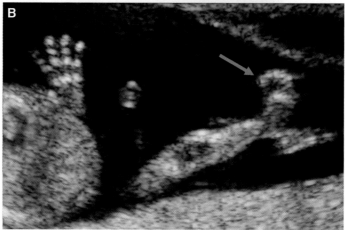

Fig. 18. Clubfeet at 12 weeks. (*A*) Transabdominal scan at 12 weeks, 4 days shows clubbed foot (*arrow*, F). (*B*) 3D surface rendered image confirms severe bilateral clubfeet (*arrow*). This was also confirmed on follow-up scans at 18 weeks.

both complicated screening and provided couples with more effective screening options. More effective screening has demonstrated that patients who traditionally were considered "high risk"-particularly patients aged 35 or older-can be at lower risk for aneuploidy and other birth defects than a 20-year-old woman who does not undergo screening. This has resulted in a clear trend in the reduction of amniocentesis for these patients, and at the same time has made screening available for younger patients who share the 2% to 3% risk of birth defects that all pregnancies carry. More effective screening translates into lower procedural-related losses of normal fetuses, and better use of resources.

The trend toward earlier detection of structural defects during the first trimester will undoubtedly continue as ultrasound resolution and 3D multiplanar ultrasound continue to improve. Conversely, a normal systematic survey at this time can be reassuring and can help to exclude a variety of major defects. Based on the presence or absence of findings, patients can then be triaged into early follow-up and possible amniocentesis at 14 to 16 weeks, or a later detailed anatomic survey at 18 to 20 weeks.

References

[1] Harper PS. Practical genetic counselling. 5th edition. Boston: Butterworth Heinemann; 1998. p. 56–70.

[2] Langdon Down J. Observations on an ethnic classification of idiots. Clin Lectures and Reports, London Hospital 1866;3:259–62.

[3] Phillips HE, McGahan JP. Intrauterine fetal cystic hygromas: sonographic detection. AJR Am J Roentgenol 1981;136(4):799–802.

[4] Toftager-Larsen K, Benzie RJ, Doran TA, et al. Alpha-fetoprotein and ultrasound scanning in the prenatal diagnosis of Turner's syndrome. Prenat Diagn 1983;3(1):35–40.

[5] Chervenak FA, Isaacson G, Blakemore KJ, et al. Fetal cystic hygroma. Cause and natural history. N Engl J Med 1983;309(14):822–5.

[6] Newman DE, Cooperberg PL. Genetics of sonographically detected intrauterine fetal cystic hygromas. J Can Assoc Radiol 1984;35(1):77–9.

[7] Brown BS, Thompson DL. Ultrasonographic features of the fetal Turner syndrome. J Can Assoc Radiol 1984;35(1):40–6.

[8] Redford DH, McNay MB, Ferguson-Smith ME, et al. Aneuploidy and cystic hygroma detectable by ultrasound. Prenat Diagn 1984;4(5):377–82.

[9] Marchese C, Savin E, Dragone E, et al. Cystic hygroma: prenatal diagnosis and genetic counselling. Prenat Diagn 1985;5(3):221–7.

[10] Garden AS, Benzie RJ, Miskin M, et al. Fetal cystic hygroma colli: antenatal diagnosis, significance, and management. Am J Obstet Gynecol 1986;154(2):221–5.

[11] Brambati B, Simoni G. Diagnosis of fetal trisomy 21 in first-trimester. Lancet 1983;1(8324):586.

[12] Gustavii B, Edvall H. First-trimester diagnosis of cystic nuchal hygroma. Acta Obstet Gynecol Scand 1984;4:383–6.

[13] Reuss A, Pijpers L, Schampers PTFN, et al. The importance of chorionic villus sampling after first-trimester diagnosis of cystic hygroma. Prenat Diagn 1987;7:299–301.

[14] Bronshtein M, Rottem S, Yoffe N, et al. First-trimester and early second-trimester diagnosis of nuchal cystic hygroma by transvaginal sonography: diverse prognosis of the septated from the nonseptated lesion. Am J Obstet Gynecol 1988; 161(1):78–82.

[15] Benacerraf BR, Barss V, Laboda LA. A sonographic sign for detection in the second-trimester of the fetus with Down's syndrome. Am J Obstet Gynecol 1985;151:1078–9.

[16] Benacerraf BR, Gelman R, Frigoletto FD. Sonographic identification of second-trimester fetuses with Down's syndrome. N Engl J Med 1987;317:1371–6.

[17] Nicolaides KH, Azar G, Byrne D, et al. Fetal nuchal translucency: ultrasound screening for chromosomal defects in first-trimester of pregnancy. BMJ 1992;304(6831):867–9.

[18] Pandya PP, Kondylios A, Hilbert L, et al. Chromosomal defects and outcome in 1015 fetuses with increased nuchal translucency. Ultrasound Obstet Gynecol 1995;5:15–9.

[19] Snijders RJM, Noble P, Sebire N, et al. UK multicentre project on assessment of risk of trisomy 21 by maternal age and fetal nuchal-translucency thickness at 10–14 weeks of gestation. Lancet 1998;352:343–6.

[20] Hyett JA, Moscoso G, Nicolaides KH. Abnormalites of the heart and great arteries in first-trimester chromosomally abnormal fetuses. Am J Med Genet 1997;69:207–16.

[21] Hyett JA, Perdu M, Sharland GK, et al. Increased nuchal translucency at 10–14 weeks of gestation as a marker for major cardiac defects. Ultrasound Obstet Gynecol 1997;10:242–6.

[22] Carvalho JS. The fetal heart or the lymphatic system or …? The quest for the etiology of increased nuchal translucency. Ultrasound Obstet Gynecol 2005;25(3):215–20.

[23] Hyett JA, Brizot ML, von Kaisenberg CS, et al. Cardiac gene expression of atrial natriuretic peptide and brain natriuretic peptide in trisomic fetuses. Obstet Gynecol 1996;87: 506–10.

[24] Matias A, Gomes C, Flack N, et al. Screening for chromosomal abnormalities at 11–14 weeks: the role of ductus venosus blood flow. Ultrasound Obstet Gynecol 1998;12:380–4.

[25] Matias A, Huggon I, Areias JC, et al. Cardiac defects in chromosomally normal fetuses with abnormal ductus venosus blood flow at 10–14 weeks. Ultrasound Obstet Gynecol 1999;14: 307–10.

[26] Chitayat D, Kalousek DK, Bamforth JS. Lymphatic abnormalities in fetuses with posterior cervical cystic hygroma. Am J Med Genet 1989;33:352–6.

[27] von Kaisenberg CS, Nicolaides KH, Brand-Saberi B. Lymphatic vessel hypoplasia in fetuses with Turner syndrome. Hum Reprod 1999;14: 823–6.

[28] Hyett J, Noble P, Sebire NJ, et al. Lethal congenital arthrogryposis presents with increased nuchal translucency at 10–14 weeks of gestation. Ultrasound Obstet Gynecol 1997;9:310–3.

[29] von Kaisenberg CS, Brand-Saberi B, Christ B, et al. Collagen Type VI gene expression in the skin of trisomy 21 fetuses. Obstet Gynecol 1998;91:319–23.

[30] von Kaisenberg CS, Krenn V, Ludwig M, et al. Morphological classification of nuchal skin in fetuses with trisomy 21, 18 and 13 at 12–18 weeks and in a trisomy 16 mouse. Anat Embryol (Berl) 1998;197:105–24.

[31] Kornman LH, Morssink LP, Beekhuis JR, et al. Nuchal translucency cannot be used as a screening test for chromosomal abnormalities in the first-trimester of pregnancy in a routine ultrasound practice. Prenat Diagn 1996;16: 797–805.

[32] Bower S, Chitty L, Bewley S, et al. First-trimester nuchal translucency screening of the general population: data from three centres [abstract]. Presented at the 27th British Congress of Obstetrics and Gynaecology. Dublin, Ireland, Royal College of Obstetrics and Gynaecology; 1995.

[33] Roberts LJ, Bewley S, Mackinson AM, et al. First-trimester fetal nuchal translucency: problems with screening the general population 1. Br J Obstet Gynaecol 1995;102:381–5.

[34] Monni G, Ibba RM, Zoppi MA. Antenatal screening for Down's syndrome. Lancet 1998; 352:1631–2.

[35] Braithwaite JM, Kadir RA, Pepera TA, et al. Nuchal translucency measurements: training of potential examiners. Ultrasound Obstet Gynecol 1996;8:192–5.

[36] Pandya PP, Altman D, Brizot ML, et al. Repeatability of measurement of fetal nuchal translucency thickness. Ultrasound Obstet Gynecol 1995;5:334–7.

[37] Pandya PP, Goldberg H, Walton B, et al. The implementation of first-trimester scanning at 10-13 weeks' gestation and the measurement of fetal nuchal translucency thickness in two maternity units. Ultrasound Obstet Gynecol 1995;5:20–5.

[38] Szabo J, Gellen J, Szemere G. First-trimester ultrasound screening for fetal aneuploidies in women over 35 and under 35 years of age. Ultrasound Obstet Gynecol 1995;5:161–3.

[39] Taipale P, Hiilesmaa V, Salonen R, et al. Increased nuchal translucency as a marker for fetal chromosomal defects. N Engl J Med 1997; 337:1654–8.

[40] Hafner E, Schuchter K, Liebhart E, et al. Results of routine fetal nuchal translucency measurement at 10–13 weeks in 4233 unselected pregnant women. Prenat Diagn 1998;18:29–34.

[41] Pajkrt E, van Lith JMM, Mol BWJ, et al. Screening for Down's syndrome by fetal nuchal translucency measurement in a general obstetric population. Ultrasound Obstet Gynecol 1998; 12:163–9.

[42] Economides DL, Whitlow BJ, Kadir R, et al. First-trimester sonographic detection of chromosomal abnormalities in an unselected population. Br J Obstet Gynaecol 1998;105:58–62.

[43] Zoppi MA, Ibba RM, Putzolu M, et al. Assessment of risk for chromosomal abnormalities at 10–14 weeks of gestation by nuchal translucency and maternal age in 5210 fetuses at a single centre. Fetal Diagn Ther 2000;15:170–3.

[44] Thilaganathan B, Sairam S, Michailidis G, et al. First-trimester nuchal translucency: effective routine screening for Down's syndrome. Br J Radiol 1999;72:946–8.

[45] Schwarzler P, Carvalho JS, Senat MV, et al. Screening for fetal aneuploidies and fetal cardiac abnormalities by nuchal translucency thickness measurement at 10–14 weeks of gestation as part of routine antenatal care in an unselected population. Br J Obstet Gynaecol 1999; 106:1029–34.

[46] Theodoropoulos P, Lolis D, Papageorgiou C, et al. Evaluation of first-trimester screening by fetal nuchal translucency and maternal age. Prenat Diagn 1988;18:133–7.

[47] Spencer K, Souter V, Tul N, et al. A screening program for trisomy 21 at 10–14 weeks using fetal nuchal translucency, maternal serum free beta-human chorionic gonadotropin and pregnancy-associated plasma protein-A. Ultrasound Obstet Gynecol 1999;13:231–7.

[48] Brizot ML, Snijders RJM, Bersinger NA, et al. Maternal serum pregnancy associated placental protein A and fetal nuchal translucency thickness for the prediction of fetal trisomies in early pregnancy. Obstet Gynecol 1994;84:918–22.

[49] Brizot ML, Snijders RJM, Butler J, et al. Maternal serum hCG and fetal nuchal translucency thickness for the prediction of fetal trisomies in the first-trimester of pregnancy. Br J Obstet Gynaecol 1995;102:1227–32.

[50] Malone FD, Ball RH, Nyberg DA, et al. FASTER Trial Research Consortium. First-trimester septated cystic hygroma: prevalence, natural history, and pediatric outcome. Obstet Gynecol 2005;106(2):288–94.

[51] Bekker MN, Haak MC, Rekoert-Hollander M, et al. Increased nuchal translucency and distended jugular lymphatic sacs on first-trimester ultrasound. Ultrasound Obstet Gynecol 2005; 25(3):239–45.

[52] Sharony R, Tepper R, Fejgin M. Fetal lateral neck cysts: the significance of associated findings. Prenat Diagn 2005;25(6):507–10.

[53] Orlandi F, Damiani G, Hallahan TW, et al. First-trimester screening for fetal aneuploidy: biochemistry and nuchal translucency. Ultrasound Obstet Gynecol 1997;10:381–6.

[54] Biagiotti R, Brizzi L, Periti E, et al. First-trimester screening for Down's syndrome using maternal serum PAPP-A and free beta-hCG in combination with fetal nuchal translucency thickness. Br J Obstet Gynaecol 1998;105:917–20.

[55] Benattar C, Audibert F, Taieb J, et al. Efficiency of ultrasound and biochemical markers for Down's syndrome risk screening. A prospective study. Fetal Diagn Ther 1999;14:112–7.

[56] De Biasio P, Siccardi M, Volpe G, et al. First-trimester screening for Down syndrome using nuchal translucency measurement with beta-hCG and PAPP-A between 10 and 13 weeks of pregnancy-the combination test. Prenat Diagn 1999;19:360–3.

[57] De Graaf IM, Parkrt E, Bilardo CM, et al. Early pregnancy screening for fetal aneuploidy with serum markers and nuchal translucency. Prenat Diagn 1999;19:458–62.

[58] Krantz DA, Hallahan TW, Orlandi F, et al. First-trimester Down syndrome screening using dried blood biochemistry and nuchal translucency. Obstet Gynecol 2000;96:207–13.

[59] Nicolaides KH. First-trimester screening for chromosomal abnormalities. Semin Perinatol 2005;29(4):190–4.

[60] Wapner R, Thom E, Simpson JL, et al. First-trimester Maternal Serum Biochemistry and Fetal Nuchal Translucency Screening (BUN) Study Group. First-trimester screening for trisomies 21 and 18. N Engl J Med 2003;349(15):1405–13.

[61] Malone FD, Canick JA, Ball RH, et al. First- and Second-Trimester Evaluation of Risk (FASTER) Research Consortium. First-trimester or second-trimester screening, or both, for Down's syndrome. N Engl J Med 2005;353(19):2001–11.

[62] Cicero S, Curcio P, Papageorghiou A, et al. Absence of nasal bone in fetuses with trisomy 21 at 11–14 weeks of gestation: an observational study. Lancet 2001;358:1665–7.

[63] Cicero S, Rembouskos G, Vandecruys H, et al. Likelihood ratio for trisomy 21 in fetuses with absent nasal bone at the 11-14 week scan. Ultrasound Obstet Gynecol 2004;23:218–23.

[64] Prefumo F, Sethna F, Sairam S, et al. First-trimester ductus venosus, nasal bones, and Down syndrome in a high-risk population. Obstet Gynecol 2005;105(6):1348–54.

[65] Otano L, Aiello H, Igarzabal L, et al. Association between first-trimester absence of fetal nasal bone on ultrasound and Down syndrome. Prenat Diagn 2002;22:930–2.

[66] Orlandi F, Bilardo CM, Campogrande M, et al. Measurement of nasal bone length at 11–14 weeks of pregnancy and its potential role in Down syndrome risk assessment. Ultrasound Obstet Gynecol 2003;22:36–9.

[67] Viora E, Masturzo B, Errange G, et al. Ultrasound evaluation of fetal nasal bone at 11 to 14 weeks in a consecutive series of 1906 fetuses. Prenat Diagn 2003;23:784–7.

[68] Zoppi MA, Ibba RM, Axiana C, et al. Absence of fetal nasal bone and aneuploidies at first-trimester nuchal translucency screening in unselected pregnancies. Prenat Diagn 2003;23:496–500.

[69] Nicolaides KH. Nuchal translucency and other first-trimester sonographic markers of chromosomal abnormalities. Am J Obstet Gynecol 2004;191:45–67.

[70] Bekker MN, Twisk JW, van Vugt JM. Reproducibility of the fetal nasal bone length measurement. J Ultrasound Med 2004;23(12):1613–8.

[71] Malone FD, Ball RH, Nyberg DA, et al. FASTER Research Consortium. First-trimester nasal bone evaluation for aneuploidy in the general population. Obstet Gynecol 2005;105(4):901.

[72] Borrell A, Gonce A, Martinez JM, et al. First-trimester screening for Down syndrome with ductus venosus Doppler studies in addition to nuchal translucency and serum markers. Prenat Diagn 2005;25(10):901–5.

[73] Faiola S, Tsoi E, Huggon IC, et al. Likelihood ratio for trisomy 21 in fetuses with tricuspid regurgitation at the 11 to 13 + 6-week scan. Ultrasound Obstet Gynecol 2005;26(1):22–7.

[74] Nicolaides KH, Spencer K, Avgidou K, et al. Multicenter study of first-trimester screening for trisomy 21 in 75 821 pregnancies: results and estimation of the potential impact of individual risk-orientated two-stage first-trimester screening. Ultrasound Obstet Gynecol 2005;25(3):221–6.

[75] Wald NJ, Watt HC, Hackshaw AK. Integrated screening for Down's syndrome based on tests performed during the first and second-trimesters. N Engl J Med 1999;341:461–7.

[76] Wald NJ, Rodeck C, Hackshaw AK, et al. SURUSS in perspective. Semin Perinatol 2005;29(4):225–35.

[77] Copel J, Bahado-Singh RO. Prenatal screening for Down's syndrome-a search for the family's values. N Engl J Med 1999;341:521–2.

[78] Benn P, Wright D, Cuckle H. Practical strategies in contingent sequential screening for Down syndrome. Prenat Diagn 2005;25(8):645–52.

[79] Wapner RJ. First-trimester screening: the BUN Study. Semin Perinatol 2005;29(4):236–9.

[80] Taipale P, Ammala M, Salonen R, et al. Two-stage ultrasonography in screening for fetal anomalies at 13–14 and 18–22 weeks of gestation. Acta Obstet Gynecol Scand 2004;83(12):1141–6.

[81] Snijders RJM, Nicolaides KH. Assessment of risks. In: Snijders RJM, Nicolaides KH, editors. Ultrasound markers for fetal chromosomal defects. Carnforth (UK): Parthenon Publishing; 1996. p. 63–120.

[82] Nyberg DA, Luthy DA, Resta RG, et al. Age-adjusted ultrasound risk assessment for fetal Down's syndrome during the second-trimester: description of the method and analysis of 142 cases. Ultrasound Obstet Gynaecol 1998;12: 8–14.

[83] Nyberg DA, Souter VL, El-Bastawissi A, et al. Isolated sonographic markers for detection of fetal Down syndrome in the second-trimester of pregnancy. J Ultrasound Med 2001;20(10): 1053–63.

[84] Malone F, Nyberg DA, Vidaver J, et al. First and second trimester evaluation of risk: The role of second trimester genetic sonography. Am J Obstet Gynecol 2004;191(6):S3.

[85] Cheng PJ, Chang SD, Shaw SW, et al. Nuchal translucency thickness in fetuses with chromosomal translocation at 11–12 weeks of gestation. Obstet Gynecol 2005;105:1058–62.

[86] Tul N, Spencer K, Noble P, et al. Screening for trisomy 18 by fetal nuchal translucency and maternal serum free beta hCG and PAPP-A at 10-14 weeks of gestation. Prenat Diagn 1999; 19:1035–42.

[87] Spencer K, Ong C, Skentou H, et al. Screening for trisomy 13 by fetal nuchal translucency and maternal serum free beta hCG and PAPP-A at 10–14 weeks of gestation. Prenat Diagn 2000;20:411–6.

[88] Spencer K, Tul N, Nicolaides KH. Maternal serum free beta hCG and PAPP-A in fetal sex chromsome defects in the first-trimester. Prenat Diagn 2000;20:390–4.

[89] Spencer K, Liao A, Skentou H, et al. Screening for triploidy by fetal nuchal translucency and maternal serum free β-hCG and PAPP-A at 10–14 weeks of gestation. Prenat Diagn 2000; 20:495–9.

[90] Souka AP, Krampl E, Bakalis S, et al. Outcome of pregnancy in chromosomally normal fetuses with increased nuchal translucency in the first-trimester. Ultrasound Obstet Gynecol 2001; 18(1):9–17.

[91] Hyett J. Does nuchal translucency have a role in fetal cardiac screening? Prenat Diagn 2004; 24(13):1130–5.

[92] McAuliffe FM, Hornberger LK, Winsor S, et al. Fetal cardiac defects and increased nuchal translucency thickness: a prospective study. Am J Obstet Gynecol 2004;191(4):1486–90.

[93] Bahado-Singh RO, Wapner R, Thom E, et al. First-trimester Maternal Serum Biochemistry and Fetal Nuchal Translucency Screening Study Group. Elevated first-trimester nuchal translucency increases the risk of congenital heart defects. Am J Obstet Gynecol 2005;192(5): 1357–61.

[94] Makrydimas G, Sotiriadis A, Huggon IC, et al. Nuchal translucency and fetal cardiac defects: a pooled analysis of major fetal echocardiography centers. Am J Obstet Gynecol 2005;192: 89–95.

[95] Gembruch U, Knopfle G, Chatterjee M, et al. First-trimester diagnosis of fetal congenital heart disease by transvaginal two-dimensional and Doppler echocardiography. Obstet Gynecol 1990;75:496–8.

[96] Bronshtein M, Siegler E, Yoffe N, et al. Prenatal diagnosis of ventricular septal defect and overriding aorta at 14 weeks' gestation, using transvaginal sonography. Prenat Diagn 1990;10: 697–702.

[97] Gembruch U, Knopfle G, Bald R, et al. Early diagnosis of fetal congenital heart disease by transvaginal echocardiography. Ultrasound Obstet Gynecol 1993;3:310–7.

[98] Achiron R, Rotstein Z, Lipitz S, et al. First-trimester diagnosis of fetal congenital heart disease by transvaginal ultrasonography. Obstet Gynecol 1994;84:69–72.

[99] Zosmer N, Souter VL, Chan CSY, et al. Early diagnosis of major cardiac defects in chromosomally normal fetuses with increased nuchal translucency. Br J Obstet Gynaecol 1999;106: 829–33.

[100] Atzei A, Gajewska K, Huggon IC, et al. Relationship between nuchal translucency thickness and prevalence of major cardiac defects in fetuses with normal karyotype. Ultrasound Obstet Gynecol 2005;26(2):154–7.

[101] Hyett JA, Perdu M, Sharland GK, et al. Using fetal nuchal translucency to screen for major congenital cardiac defects at 10–14 weeks of gestation: population based cohort study. BMJ 1999;318:81–5.

[102] Carvahlo JS, Moscoso G, Ville Y. First-trimester transabdominal fetal echocardiography. Lancet 1998;351:1023–7.

[103] Souka AP, Von Kaisenberg CS, Hyett JA, et al. Increased nuchal translucency with normal karyotype. Am J Obstet Gynecol 2005;192:1005–21.

[104] Hiippala A, Eronen M, Taipale P, et al. Fetal nuchal translucency and normal chromosomes: a long-term follow-up study. Ultrasound Obstet Gynecol 2001;18:18–22.

[105] Sebire NJ, Snijders RJM, Hughes K, et al. Screening for trisomy 21 in twin pregnancies by maternal age and fetal nuchal translucency thickness at 10-14 weeks of gestation. Br J Obstet Gynaecol 1996;103:999–1003.

[106] Bush MC, Malone FD. Down syndrome screening in twins. Clin Perinatol 2005;32(2): 373–86.

[107] Sebire NJ, Hughes K, D'Ercole C, et al. Increased fetal nuchal translucency at 10–14 weeks as a predictor of severe twin-to-twin transfusion syndrome. Ultrasound Obstet Gynecol 1997; 10:86–9.

[108] Shalev E, Zalele Y, Ben Ami M, et al. First-trimester ultrasonic diagnosis of twin reversed arterial perfusion sequence. Prenat Diagn 1992;2: 21–2.

[109] Langlotz H, Sauerbrei E, Murray S. Transvaginal Doppler sonographic diagnosis of an acardiac

twin at 12 week gestation. J Ultrasound Med 1991;10:175–9.

[110] van Eyndhoven HW, ter Brugge H. The first-trimester ultrasonographic diagnosis of dicephalus conjoined twins. Acta Obstet Gynecol Scand 1998;77:464–6.

[111] Tongsong T, Chanprapaph P, Pongsatha S. First-trimester diagnosis of conjoined twins: a report of three cases. Ultrasound Obstet Gynecol 1999; 14:434–7.

[112] Bonilla-Musoles F, Raga F, Bonilla F Jr, et al. Early diagnosis of conjoined twins using two-dimensional color Doppler and three-dimensional ultrasound. J Natl Med Assoc 1998;90:552–6.

[113] Goldberg Y, Ben-Shlomo I, Weiner E, et al. First-trimester diagnosis of conjoined twins in a triplet pregnancy after IVF and ICSI: case report. Hum Reprod 2000;15:1413–5.

[114] Hill LM. The sonographic detection of early first-trimester conjoined twins. Prenat Diagn 1997;17:961–3.

[115] Lam YH, Sin SY, Lam C, et al. Prenatal sonographic diagnosis of conjoined twins in the first-trimester: two case reports. Ultrasound Obstet Gynecol 1998;11:289–91.

[116] Maymon R, Halperin R, Weinraub Z, et al. Three-dimensional transvaginal sonography of conjoined twins at 10 weeks: a case report. Ultrasound Obstet Gynecol 1998;11:292–4.

[117] Meizner I, Levy A, Katz M, et al. Early ultrasonic diagnosis of conjoined twins. Harefuah 1993; 124:741–4.

[118] Schmidt W, Heberling D, Kubli F. Antepartum ultrasonographic diagnosis of conjoined twins in early pregnancy. Am J Obstet Gynecol 1981; 139:961–3.

[119] Efrat Z, Akinfenwa OO, Nicolaides KH. First-trimester determination of fetal gender by ultrasound. Ultrasound Obstet Gynecol 1999;13: 305–7.

[120] Inman V, Saunders JB de CM. The ossification of the human frontal bone. J Anat 1937;71: 383–94.

[121] Kennedy KA, Flick KJ, Thurmond AS. First-trimester diagnosis of exencephaly. Am J Obstet Gynecol 1990;162:461–3.

[122] Johnson SP, Sebire NJ, Snijders RJ, et al. Ultrasound screening for anencephaly at 10–14 postmenstrual weeks. Ultrasound Obstet Gynecol 1997;9:14–6.

[123] Bronshtein M, Timor-Tritsch I, Rottem S. Early detection of fetal anomalies. In: Timor-Tritsch I, Rottem S, editors. Transvaginal sonography. New York: Chapman & Hall; 1991. p. 327–71.

[124] Gonzalez-Gomez F, Salamanca A, Padilla MC, et al. Alobar holoprosencephalic embryo detected via transvaginal sonography. Eur J Obstet Gynecol Reprod Biol 1992;47:266–70.

[125] Turner CD, Silva S, Jeanty P. Prenatal diagnosis of alobar holoprosencephaly at 10 postmenstrual weeks. Ultrasound Obstet Gynecol 1999; 13:360–2.

[126] Baxi L, Warren W, Collins MH, et al. Early detection of caudal regression syndrome with transvaginal scanning. Obstet Gynecol 1990; 75:486–9.

[127] Nicolaides KH, Campbell S, Gabbe SG, et al. Ultrasound screening for spina bifida: cranial and cerebellar signs. Lancet 1986;2:72–4.

[128] Campbell J, Gilbert WM, Nicolaides KH, et al. Ultrasound screening for spina bifida: cranial and cerebellar signs in a high-risk population. Obstet Gynecol 1987;70:247–50.

[129] Sebire NJ, Noble PL, Thorpe-Beeston JG, et al. Presence of the 'lemon' sign in fetuses with spina bifida at the 10–14-week scan. Ultrasound Obstet Gynecol 1997;10:403–5.

[130] Bernard JP, Suarez B, Rambaud C, et al. Prenatal diagnosis of neural tube defect before 12 weeks' gestation: direct and indirect ultrasonographic semeiology. Ultrasound Obstet Gynecol 1997; 10:406–9.

[131] Blumenfeld Z, Siegler E, Bronshtein M. The early diagnosis of neural tube defects. Prenat Diagn 1993;13:863–71.

[132] Merz E, Weber G, Bahlmann F, et al. Application of transvaginal and abdominal three-dimensional ultrasound for the detection or exclusion of malformations of the fetal face. Ultrasound Obstet Gynecol 1997;9:237–43.

[133] Nyberg D, Mahoney B, Kramer D. Paranasal echogenic mass: sonographic sign of bilateral complete cleft lip and palate before 20 menstrual weeks. Radiology 1992;184(3): 757–9.

[134] Bronshtein M, Zimmer E, Gershoni-Baruch R, et al. First- and second -trimester diagnosis of fetal ocular defects and associated anomalies: report of eight cases. Obstet Gynecol 1991;77: 443–9.

[135] Feldman E, Shalev E, Weiner E, et al. Microphthalmia-prenatal ultrasonic diagnosis: a case report. Prenat Diagn 1985;5:205–7.

[136] Jeanty P, Dramaix-Wilmet M, Van Gansbeke D, et al. Fetal ocular biometry by ultrasound. Radiology 1982;143:513–6.

[137] Monteagudo A, Timor-Tritsch IE, Friedman AH, et al. Autosomal dominant cataracts of the fetus: early detection by transvaginal ultrasound. Ultrasound Obstet Gynecol 1996;8:104–8.

[138] Zimmer E, Bronshtein M, Ophir E, et al. Sonographic diagnosis of fetal congenital cataracts. Prenat Diagn 1993;13:503–11.

[139] Dolkart LA, Reimers FT. Transvaginal fetal echocardiography in early pregnancy: normative data. Am J Obstet Gynecol 1991;165: 688–91.

[140] Bronshtein M, Siegler E, Eshcoli Z, et al. Transvaginal ultrasound measurements of the fetal heart at 11 to 17 weeks. Am J Perinatol 1992; 9:38–42.

[141] Guzman ER. Early prenatal diagnosis of gastroschisis with transvaginal ultrasonography. Am J Obstet Gynecol 1990;162:1253–4.

[142] Kushnir O, Izquierdo L, Vigil D, et al. Early transvaginal sonographic diagnosis of gastroschisis. J Clin Ultrasound 1990;18:194–7.

[143] Fleming AD, Vintzileos AM, Rodis JF, et al. Diagnosis of fetal ectopia cordis by transvaginal ultrasound. J Ultrasound Med 1991;10:413–5.

[144] Bennett TL, Burlbaw J, Drake CK, et al. Diagnosis of ectopia cordis at 12 postmenstrual weeks using transabdominal ultrasonography with color flow Doppler. J Ultrasound Med 1991;10:695–6.

[145] Forrester MB, Merz RD. Epidemiology of abdominal wall defects, Hawaii, 1986–1997. Teratology 1999;60:117–23.

[146] Becker R, Runkel S, Entezami M. Prenatal diagnosis of body stalk anomaly at 9 weeks. case report. Fetal Diagn Ther 2000;15:301–3.

[147] Cyr DR, Mack LA, Schoenecker SA, et al. Bowel migration in the normal fetus: US detection. Radiology 1986;161:119–21.

[148] Curtis JA, Watson L. Sonographic diagnosis of omphalocele in the first-trimester of fetal gestation. J Ultrasound Med 1988;7:97–100.

[149] Nyberg DA, Fitzsimmons J, Mack LA, et al. Chromosomal abnormalities in fetuses with omphalocele. Significance of omphalocele contents. J Ultrasound Med 1989;8:299–308.

[150] Benacerraf BR, Saltzman DH, Estroff JA, et al. Abnormal karyotype of fetuses with omphalocele: prediction based on omphalocele contents. Obstet Gynecol 1990;75:317–9.

[151] Pagliano M, Mossetti M, Ragno P. Echographic diagnosis of omphalocele in the first-trimester of pregnancy. J Clin Ultrasound 1990;18:658–60.

[152] Brown DL, Emerson DS, Shulman LP, et al. Sonographic diagnosis of omphalocele during 10th week of gestation. AJR Am J Roentgenol 1989;153:825–6.

[153] Gray DL, Martin CM, Crane JP. Differential diagnosis of first-trimester ventral wall defect. J Ultrasound Med 1989;8:255–8.

[154] Moore K. The urogenital system. In: Moore K, editor. The developing human. Clinically oriented embryology. Philadelphia: WB Saunders Company; 1988. p. 246–85.

[155] Rosati P, Guariglia L. Transvaginal sonographic assessment of the fetal urinary tract in early pregnancy. Ultrasound Obstet Gynecol 1996;7:95–100.

[156] Green JJ, Hobbins JC. Abdominal ultrasound examination of the first-trimester fetus. Am J Obstet Gynecol 1988;159:165–75.

[157] Bronshtein M, Kushnir O, Ben-Rafael Z, et al. Transvaginal sonographic measurement of fetal kidneys in the first-trimester of pregnancy. J Clin Ultrasound 1990;18:299–301.

[158] Bronshtein M, Bar-Hava I, Blumenfeld Z. Clues and pitfalls in the early prenatal diagnosis of 'late onset' infantile polycystic kidney. Prenat Diagn 1992;12:293–8.

[159] Bronshtein M, Bar-Hava I, Blumenfeld Z. Differential diagnosis of the nonvisualized fetal urinary bladder by transvaginal sonography in the early second-trimester. Obstet Gynecol 1993;82:490–3.

[160] Zimmer EZ, Bronshtein M. Fetal intra-abdominal cysts detected in the first and early second-trimester by transvaginal sonography. J Clin Ultrasound 1991;19:564–7.

[161] Stiller RJ. Early ultrasonic appearance of fetal bladder outlet obstruction. Am J Obstet Gynecol 1989;160:584–5.

[162] Liao AW, Sebire NJ, Geerts L, et al. Megacystis at 10–14 weeks of gestation: chromosomal defects and outcome according to bladder length. Ultrasound Obstet Gynecol 2003;21(4):338–41.

[163] Favre R, Kohler M, Gasser B, et al. Early fetal megacystis between 11 and 15 weeks. Ultrasound Obstet Gynecol 1999;14:402–6.

[164] Moore K. The limbs. In: Moore K, editor. The developing human. Clinically oriented embryology. Philadelphia: WB Saunders Company; 1988. p. 355–63.

[165] Timor Tritsch IE, Farine D, Rosen MG. A close look at early embryonic development with the high-frequency transvaginal transducer. Am J Obstet Gynecol 1988;159:676–81.

[166] Mahoney B. Ultrasound evaluation of the fetal musculoskeletal system. In: Callen P, editor. Ultrasonography in obstetrics and gynecology. Philadelphia: WB Saunders Company; 1994. p. 254–90.

[167] Timor-Tritsch IE, Monteagudo A, Peisner DB. High-frequency transvaginal sonographic examination for the potential malformation assessment of the 9-week to 14-week fetus. J Clin Ultrasound 1992;20:231–8.

[168] Bronshtein M, Keret D, Deutsch M, et al. Transvaginal sonographic detection of skeletal anomalies in the first and early second-trimesters. Prenat Diagn 1993;13:597–601.

[169] D'Ottavio G, Tamaro LF, Mandruzzato G. Early prenatal ultrasonographic diagnosis of osteogenesis imperfecta: a case report. Am J Obstet Gynecol 1993;169:384–5.

[170] DiMaio MS, Barth R, Koprivnikar KE, et al. First-trimester prenatal diagnosis of osteogenesis imperfecta Type II by DNA analysis and sonography. Prenat Diagn 1993;13:589–96.

[171] Brons JT, van der Harten HJ, Wladimiroff JW, et al. Prenatal ultrasonographic diagnosis of osteogenesis imperfecta. Am J Obstet Gynecol 1988;159:176–81.

[172] Stephens JD, Filly RA, Callen PW, et al. Prenatal diagnosis of osteogenesis imperfecta Type II by real-time ultrasound. Hum Genet 1983;64:191–3.

[173] Sepulveda W, Romero R, Pryde PG, et al. Prenatal diagnosis of sirenomelus with color Doppler ultrasonography. Am J Obstet Gynecol 1994;170:1377–9.

[174] Sepulveda W, Corral E, Sanchez J, et al. Sirenomelia sequence versus renal agenesis: prenatal
differentiation with power Doppler ultrasound. Ultrasound Obstet Gynecol 1998;11:
445–9.

[175] van Zalen-Sprock MM, van Vugt JM, van der
Harten JJ, et al. Early second-trimester
diagnosis of sirenomelia. Prenat Diagn 1995;
15:171–7.

[176] Valenzano M, Paoletti R, Rossi A, et al. Sirenomelia. Pathological features, antenatal ultrasonographic clues, and a review of current
embryogenic theories. Hum Reprod Update
1999;5:82–6.

RADIOLOGIC
CLINICS
OF NORTH AMERICA

Radiol Clin N Am 44 (2006) 863–877

ELSEVIER
SAUNDERS

Imaging of Pelvic Pain in the First Trimester of Pregnancy

Aimee D. Eyvazzadeh, MD[a], Deborah Levine, MD[b],*

The noninvasive nature, safety, and reliability of ultrasonography make it the diagnostic method of choice for pregnant patients who have pelvic pain. Sonography provides information that allows for diagnosis of both pregnancy-related pain, such as a ruptured ectopic pregnancy, miscarriage, or threatened abortion; and may be useful in the diagnosis of pain unrelated to pregnancy, such as that seen in appendicitis and nephrolithiasis.

Normal pregnancy

Because of hormonal changes, rapid growth of the uterus, and increased blood flow, "crampy" pelvic pain is common in early pregnancy. For the primapara, this pain can be quite worrisome. It is common for pregnant patients to present with pain in the first trimester and have normal findings on sonography. The first sonographic demonstration of early pregnancy is the intradecidual sign [Fig. 1] [1–3]. This is visualized as a discrete hypoechoic fluid collection with an echogenic rim that is eccentrically located in the endometrial cavity, and deviates the endometrial stripe. This is seen at 4.5 to 5 weeks of gestation [3]. Because small endometrial fluid collections can simulate the intradecidual sign, care should be taken to ensure that the collection has a well-defined echogenic rim, is just

This article was originally published in *Ultrasound Clinics* 1:2, April 2006.
[a] Department of Obstetrics and Gynecology, Beth Israel Deaconess Medical Center, 330 Brookline Avenue, Boston, MA 02215, USA
[b] Department of Radiology, Beth Israel Deaconess Medical Center, 330 Brookline Avenue, Boston, MA 02215, USA
* Corresponding author.
E-mail address: dlevine@bidmc.harvard.edu (D. Levine).

doi:10.1016/j.rcl.2006.10.015

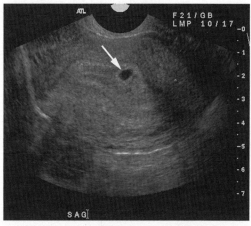

Fig. 1. Normal early pregnancy. Sagittal view of the uterus at 4 1/2 weeks gestational age shows an intra-decidual sign with a small sac (*arrow*) eccentrically located in the endometrium.

beneath the central endometrial echo, and has an unchanging appearance [1]. It is prudent to obtain follow-up in patients at high risk for ectopic pregnancy or patients who have symptoms in order to ensure that an intrauterine pregnancy is present.

Slightly later the decidua capsularis and decidua vera are seen as two distinct hyperechoic layers surrounding the early gestational sac; this is known as the double decidual sac sign [4]. The yolk sac is the next structure to be visualized. It appears as a small hyperechoic ring within the gestational sac, and is present at 5.5 weeks [Fig. 2]. Finally, the embryo can be seen adjacent to the yolk sac. Cardiac activity can usually be observed whenever an embryonic pole is seen, but should be visualized by the time the embryonic pole is 5 mm [5,6].

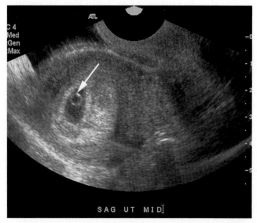

Fig. 2. Normal early pregnancy. Sagittal view of the uterus at 5 1/2 weeks gestational age shows a yolk sac (*arrow*) within the intrauterine gestational sac.

Subchorionic hemorrhage

Subchorionic hemorrhage is seen on ultrasound in 4% to 22% of patients who have symptoms of pain and bleeding in early pregnancy [7]. It is caused by a partial detachment of the trophoblast from the uterine wall. On ultrasound the placental margin is displaced by anechoic or heterogeneous hypoechoic material [8]. Small echogenic structures can be found in such areas, likely due to blood clots. Because the hematoma can dissect in the potential space between the chorion and endometrial cavity, it may be visualized separate from the placenta. Because it typically conforms to the shape of the uterus, it usually has a falciform shape [Fig. 3]. A small collection likely has no clinical significance, whereas moderate or large subchorionic hematomas have a poorer prognosis [9]. Seventy percent of subchorionic hematomas resolve spontaneously by the end of the second trimester [10]. As in all early pregnancy assessments, demonstration of cardiac activity is crucial in determining prognosis.

Spontaneous abortion

First-trimester spontaneous abortion occurs in 10% to 12% of clinically recognized pregnancies [11]. Pain may be constant or intermittent and crampy over the uterus or lower back. Most women with spontaneous abortion experience vaginal bleeding. Up to 25% of all pregnant women bleed some time during pregnancy, with about half of them eventually undergoing miscarriage. The term "threatened abortion" is used to define bleeding in the first 20 weeks of pregnancy with a closed internal os. Ultrasound in the case of a threatened abortion is used to detect an intrauterine pregnancy and to determine if a live embryo or fetus is present. The landmarks for normal pregnancy help to distinguish between a normal early intrauterine pregnancy and a miscarriage. To ensure high specificity in our diagnosis of spontaneous abortion, the authors use generous thresholds: visualization of a yolk sac by the time the gestational sac has a mean sac diameter of 13 mm, visualization of an embryo by the time the mean sac diameter is 18 mm, and visualization of cardiac activity by the time the embryonic pole is 5 mm [12]. Between 6.5 to 10 weeks of gestation, the length of the amniotic cavity is similar to that of the embryo. At times a failed early pregnancy will present as an "empty amnion sign" [13] [Fig. 4].

In addition to the absolute criteria mentioned above, sonographic findings in spontaneous abortion include a thin decidual reaction (less than 2 mm), weak decidual amplitude, irregular contour of the sac, absent double decidual sac sign, and low position of the sac.

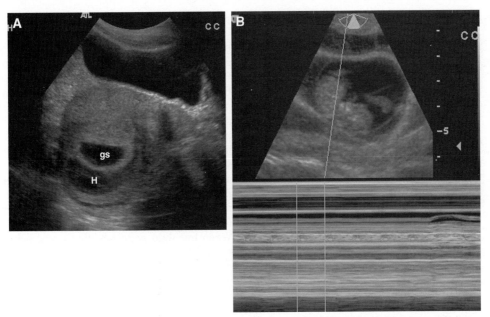

Fig. 3. Subchorionic hematoma at 10 weeks gestational age. (*A*) Transabdominal sagittal image shows an intra-uterine gestational sac (*gs*) with a subchorionic hematoma (*H*). (*B*) Transvaginal view with m-mode shows fetal pole with normal cardiac activity.

Molar pregnancy

Molar pregnancy can be associated with pelvic pain because of either the rapid change in size of the uterus, the size of the associated theca lutein cysts,

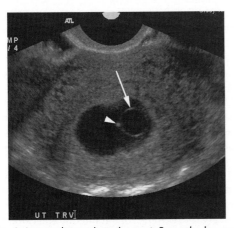

Fig. 4. Incomplete miscarriage at 8 weeks by menstrual dates. A prior sonogram had shown a live embryo. Transvaginal image of the uterus shows an intrauterine gestational sac with mean sac diameter of 22 mm. An amnion (*arrow*) is present that measures 10 mm. A residual 1 mm embryonic pole is present (*arrowhead*). No yolk sac was visualized. Even without the history of a prior sonogram demonstrating a live pregnancy, a miscarriage can be diagnosed because the amnion is much larger than the residual embryonic pole.

or torsion of the ovaries caused by the theca lutein cysts [Fig. 5]. The classic sonographic appearance of a complete mole has multiple cystic spaces representing hydropic villi; however, the size of the villi is directly proportional to gestational age [14], and early molar pregnancies frequently do not have the typical sonographic appearance [15]. Other appearances that can be seen in the first trimester include an intrauterine anechoic fluid collection similar to a gestational sac, a fluid collection with a complex echogenic mass similar to an edematous placenta, a heterogeneously thickened endometrium, and echogenic fluid-fluid levels within the endometrium [15].

Corpus luteum

The corpus luteum is the most common adnexal mass in pregnancy, and is a common cause of pelvic pain. The pain is lateralized to the side of the cyst. Pain can be due to the size of the cyst, bleeding within the cyst, torsion, or rupture. The cyst is typically less than 6 cm in diameter, but may be larger. There is typically posterior through transmission because of the cystic composition. The internal echotexture varies, depending on the stage of hemorrhage and the amount of fluid within the cyst. This is best appreciated with transvaginal scanning. The diagnosis of a hemorrhagic cyst can be made with the presence of fibrin strands, a retracting clot, septations, and wall irregularity [16,17]. The

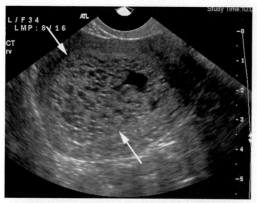

Fig. 5. Molar pregnancy at 10 weeks gestational age in patient with pelvic pain. Sagittal transvaginal image shows the endometrial cavity (*arrows*) to be distended with echogenic material with multiple small cysts compatible with a molar pregnancy. Human chorionic gonadotropin level was 42,000.

wall of the cyst may appear thick or thin, ranging from 2 to 22 mm [Fig. 6]. The corpus luteum is a very vascular structure, and typically a ring of color flow can be demonstrated [Fig. 7] [18]. It is important to recognize that this flow is a normal finding, so as not to mistake a corpus luteum for an ectopic pregnancy.

If a hemorrhagic corpus luteum cyst is the cause of the patient's pain, it should be tender to direct pressure using the transvaginal probe. If it is pain-free, another source for the patient's pelvic pain should be sought.

Hemoperitoneum

Echogenic fluid suggests hemoperitoneum. When echogenic fluid is visualized in a patient who has

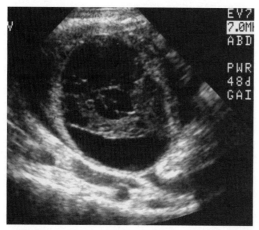

Fig. 6. Transverse transvaginal image of a hemorrhagic cyst. Note the strands of internal density that have a "cobweb" appearance.

positive β-hCG results, this has a positive predictive value (86%–93%) in the diagnosis of ectopic pregnancy [19], and may be the only endovaginal sonographic finding [20]; however, a ruptured hemorrhagic corpus luteum cyst can also result in hemoperitoneum [Fig. 8]. If the patient is clinically unstable, differentiating between a ruptured ectopic and a ruptured hemorrhagic corpus luteum is unimportant, because in either case a laparotomy is indicated. In unstable patients who have demonstration of hemoperitoneum, the sonographic examination may not demonstrate an ectopic pregnancy. In the clinically stable patient it is more important to carefully examine the adnexa to determine if an ectopic pregnancy is present. When free fluid is documented in the pelvis, it is helpful to obtain images of the kidneys to assess whether a large amount of hemoperitoneum is present [Fig. 9].

Ectopic pregnancy

Symptoms of an ectopic pregnancy are pelvic and abdominal pain and amenorrhea. Vaginal spotting or bleeding may be present. In a 5-year review of 98 cases who underwent surgery for ectopic, Aboud [21] showed that the most common presenting symptoms were pain (in 97%), followed by vaginal bleeding (in 79%), with the most frequent physical findings being abdominal tenderness (in 91%) and adnexal tenderness (in 54%). The combination of ultrasound and hCG level is the best way to diagnose an ectopic pregnancy. More than 1 in every 100 pregnancies in the United States is ectopic [22]. The incidence has increased fourfold from 1970 to 1992 [22]. Some causes include a higher incidence of salpingitis and an increased use of assisted reproductive techniques [23].

Patients typically present at about 5 to 6 weeks gestational age. Because menstrual dates are often inaccurate, however, an early gestational age by dates should not influence the diligence taken to diagnose an ectopic pregnancy.

The possibility of an ectopic pregnancy is low if a gestational sac is clearly documented within the uterine cavity. The incidence of heterotopic pregnancy (the occurrence of intrauterine and extrauterine pregnancy) ranges from 1/2,100 to 1/30,000 [24,25]. Of importance, the incidence is as high as 2.9% in the assisted fertilization population [26,27]. Therefore, although visualization of an intrauterine gestation is crucial, careful attention to the adnexa is always important.

Ectopic pregnancy should be suspected in patients who present with a positive pregnancy test with absence of an intrauterine pregnancy on ultrasound. In general, an intrauterine gestational sac

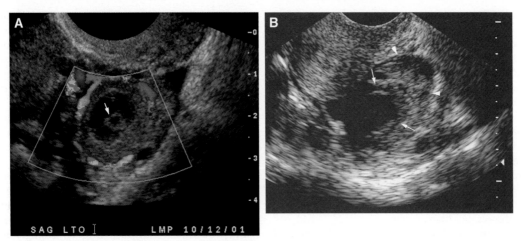

Fig. 7. Ring of flow on hemorrhagic cyst. (*A*) Sagittal transvaginal color Doppler image of 2 cm thick-walled hemorrhagic cyst in a pregnant patient. Note the central fibrin stand mimicking a yolk sac (*arrow*). Note the ring-of-fire appearance to the cyst. (*B*) Transverse, transvaginal image of the same patient in (*A*), showing that the mass (*arrows*) is located within the ovary (*arrowheads*). Additional images (not shown) demonstrated an intrauterine gestational sac with yolk sac. (*From* Swire MN, Castro-Aragon I, Levine D. Various sonographic appearances of the hemorrhagic corpus luteum cyst. Ultrasound Q 2004;20:49; with permission.)

is expected to be visualized when β-hCG is 1000 mIU/ml (Second International Standard,) or 2000 mIU/ml international reference preparation (IRP) [28,29]. It should be emphasized that the majority of studies of b-hCG in early pregnancy evaluated normal early pregnancy, and described an intrauterine gestational sac as any collection of fluid in the endometrial cavity. Small fluid collections of 2 mm without a decidual reaction were considered sufficient to describe an early gestational sac. It should be noted that this type of fluid collection can be caused by a decidual cyst or even a pseudo-sac, and therefore may not represent a normal intrauterine pregnancy; however, these values are helpful in triaging patients. When β-hCG is below the discriminatory zone (2000 mIU/mL, IRP) and no intrauterine gestation is present, the diagnosis could be an early intrauterine pregnancy, a miscarriage, or an ectopic pregnancy, and therefore close follow-up is indicated [30]. When the β-hCG value is above the discriminatory zone, one can expect to

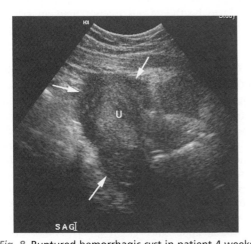

Fig. 8. Ruptured hemorrhagic cyst in patient 4 weeks pregnant with pelvic pain. Sagittal view of the uterus shows hemorrhage (*arrows*) around the uterus (U). No intrauterine gestational sac was seen. Because of continued pain and bleeding, the patient underwent laparotomy. A ruptured hemorrhagic cyst was found. Follow-up sonogram demonstrated a live intrauterine pregnancy.

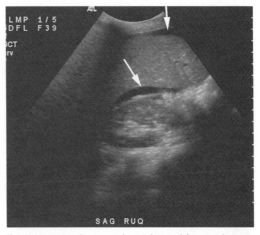

Fig. 9. Hemoperitoneum in patient with ectopic pregnancy. Oblique sagittal view of right upper quadrant in patient with pelvic pain in the first trimester shows fluid (*arrows*) around the liver and kidneys, consistent with a large amount of hemoperitoneum.

see an intrauterine gestational sac; however, even without visualization of a sac there could still be a very early normal intrauterine pregnancy. Technical quality of the examination, presence of fibroids, intrauterine contraceptive devices, large hemorrhage, and multiple gestation may contribute to nonvisualization of an early sac [30–32]; however, none of these factors may be present, and follow-up may still reveal a normal early pregnancy [30]. Because of this, and because stable patients can be watched rather than treated [33–35], it is reasonable to follow stable patients who have a nonvisualized gestational sac with serial β-hCG and ultrasound rather than immediately treating with methotrexate or laparotomy.

A normal pregnancy shows a doubling time of the β-hCG value of 2 days (range 1.2–2.2 days) [36]. This doubling time is increased in ectopic pregnancy. If the β-hCG values rise abnormally (<60% increase over 48 hours and not steadily declining), the patient is presumed to have an ectopic pregnancy.

The most common location for ectopic pregnancy is in the fallopian tubes, occurring in up to 97% of the cases. Of these, 75% to 80% are located in the ampullary region, 10% in the isthmic portion, 5% in the fimbrial portion, and 2% to 4% in the interstitial portion. Uncommon locations include the ovary, abdomen, cervix, and uterine scars [37,38]. Because most ectopic pregnancies are located within the tubes, it is important to scan above and below the ovaries and between the uterus and ovaries.

Sonographic diagnosis of ectopic pregnancy

Endometrial findings

Small fluid collections without an echogenic rim can be present. These decidual cysts are typically located at the junction of the endometrium with the myometrium, and were originally reported as being highly specific for ectopic pregnancy [39], but are now known to be neither specific nor sensitive [40,41]. When fluid is seen centrally in the endometrial cavity, this is termed a "pseudosac" [Fig. 10]. This fluid collection represents blood in the endometrial cavity, which can be present in both intrauterine and ectopic pregnancies. The pseudosac has only one layer corresponding to the endometrial decidual reaction, compared with the double decidual sac sign seen in early intrauterine pregnancy [4].

Adnexal findings

The most specific finding for ectopic pregnancy is the presence of a live extrauterine pregnancy [Fig. 11]; however, this pathognomonic sign is present only in only 8% to 26% of ectopic pregnancies on transvaginal sonogram [42]. The next most specific sign is an extrauterine gestational sac containing a yolk sac, with or without an embryo [see Fig. 10] [19]; however, care should be taken not to confuse a hemorrhagic cyst with debris mimicking a yolk sac or embryo [see Fig. 7].

An extra-ovarian tubal ring is 40% to 68% sensitive for ectopic pregnancy [see Fig. 10] [43,44]. Slightly less specific but most common is a complex adnexal mass separate from the ovary [19,20,31, 43–55]. These should be distinguished from a hemorrhagic corpus luteum cyst arising from the ovary. The transvaginal transducer can be used "real-time" to determine if the echogenic ring moves with or is independent of, the ovary. Another sonographic finding that can help distinguish the corpus luteum from the adnexal ring of an ectopic pregnancy is the relative echogenicity of the wall of the corpus luteum compared with that of a tubal ectopic and of the endometrium. The wall of a corpus luteum is less echogenic when compared with the wall of the tubal ring associated with an ectopic pregnancy, and is less echogenic compared with the endometrium [56,57]. If the diagnosis of an adherent ectopic pregnancy or an exophytic ovarian cyst cannot be confirmed and the patient is stable, a follow-up examination is reasonable, because an intrauterine pregnancy may be seen on follow-up, and a hemorrhagic cyst is expected to undergo evolution.

The least specific finding of ectopic pregnancy is the presence of any adnexal mass other than a simple cyst. Even a complex cyst in the ovary is more likely to be the corpus luteum than an ectopic pregnancy.

Use of color Doppler in diagnosis of ectopic pregnancy

Using color Doppler flow, uterine or extrauterine sites of vascular color can be identified in a characteristic placental shape, the so-called "ring-of-fire" pattern, and a high-velocity, low-impedance flow pattern may also be identified that is compatible with placental perfusion [58]. A ring of fire has been described as characterizing the appearance of flow around an ectopic pregnancy; however, the corpus luteum is also very vascular and can have a similar appearance [see Fig. 7] [59,60]. Color Doppler is most helpful when an extra ovarian mass has not yet been found, because use of Doppler may allow for detection of an ectopic surrounded by loops of bowel. Luteal flow can be helpful in identifying an ectopic, because about 90% of ectopic pregnancies occur on the same side as luteal flow [61].

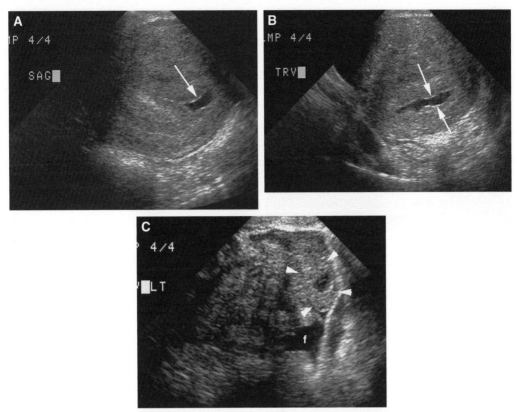

Fig. 10. Pseudosac in patient with ectopic pregnancy at 5 weeks gestational age. Transvaginal sagittal (*A*) and transverse (*B*) images show fluid (*arrows*) centrally located within the endometrial cavity. Oblique image in the left adnexa (*C*) shows a ringlike mass (*arrowheads*) with a faint yolk sac and some free fluid (*f*). The mass was separate from the left ovary (not shown). A left-sided ectopic pregnancy was confirmed at laparotomy.

Interstitial pregnancy

Interstitial pregnancies represent 2% to 4% of ectopic pregnancies [62]. These pregnancies are associated with a higher morbidity and mortality than other tubal pregnancies [63]. Although some term these "cornual pregnancies," this term is best used if pregnancy occurs in a bicornuate uterus. The high morbidity from these pregnancies is caused by the fact that the interstitial portion of the tube dilates more freely and painlessly than the rest of the tube, leading to later clinical presentation than the typical ectopic pregnancy, and the potential for massive hemorrhage. Rupture occurs later in interstitial ectopics, usually between 8 and 16 weeks. Because the implantation site may be located between the ovarian and uterine arteries, rupture in this area may prove fatal [64].

The diagnosis is suggested when what appears to be an intrauterine pregnancy is visualized high in the fundus and is not surrounded in all planes by 5 mm of myometrium [Fig. 12] [44,65]. These can be treated with laparotomy, systemic methotrexate [66], or transvaginal, sonographically guided injection of potassium chloride [67].

Cervical ectopic pregnancy

Cervical ectopic pregnancy occurs in fewer than 1% of all ectopics [68,69]. The sonographic diagnosis is made when a gestational sac with peritrophoblastic flow or a live embryo is identified within the cervix. When a gestational sac with a yolk sac or embryo is seen within the cervix without a heartbeat, the differential diagnosis includes spontaneous abortion and cervical ectopic. Follow-up scanning allows for differentiation; in cases of ectopic pregnancy the sac does not change in position, whereas in spontaneous abortion, the sac shape and position will change. Patients who have cervical ectopics tend to bleed profusely because the cervix does not have contractile tissue. Therefore treatment by dilatation and curettage is more risky than treatment of an intrauterine pregnancy. Because of these risks, in the past cervical ectopics were often treated with hysterectomy. Newer conservative therapies include sonographically guided local potassium chloride injection [67,70,71], systemic or local methotrexate [71–74], or preoperative uterine artery embolization before dilatation and evacuation [71,75].

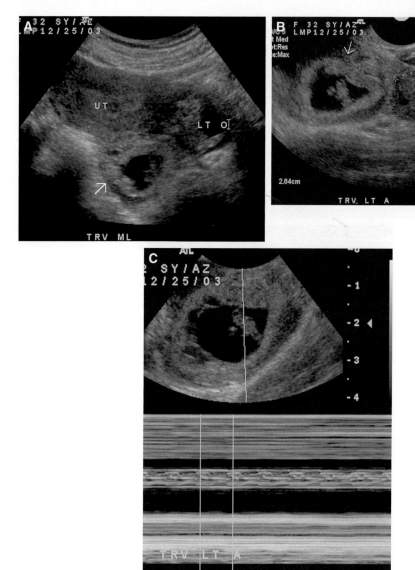

Fig. 11. Live ectopic pregnancy. (A) Transverse transabdominal image shows a left- sided gestational sac (*arrow*) adjacent to the uterus (*UT*), clearly separate from the left ovary (*LT O*). (B) Transverse transvaginal image shows the ectopic pregnancy adjacent to the left ovary. (C) M-Mode demonstrates cardiac activity.

Scar pregnancy

Scars in the uterus can be sites for implantation of pregnancy. Cesarean section scar pregnancy is being increasingly reported [76]. There is complete embedding of the gestational sac in the myometrium. The myometrium between the bladder and the sac becomes thinner or disappears because of distension of the sac. Only the thin, serosal layer is apparent. Criteria used for diagnosis are an empty uterus, empty cervical canal, and development of the sac in the anterior part of the lower uterine segment [Fig. 13] [77]. Current non- and minimally invasive treatments include sonographically guided

methotrexate or potassium chloride injection [67,78], or intramuscular methotrexate [79]. Definitive treatment of a cesarean scar pregnancy is by laparotomy and hysterotomy, with repair of the accompanying uterine scar dehiscence [80]. Other procedures that scar the uterus put the patient at increased risk for scar pregnancy. For example, a pregnancy can implant in a myomectomy scar [60].

Ovarian and abdominal ectopic pregnancy

Ovarian pregnancies usually appear as an ovarian cyst with a wide, echogenic outside ring. A yolk

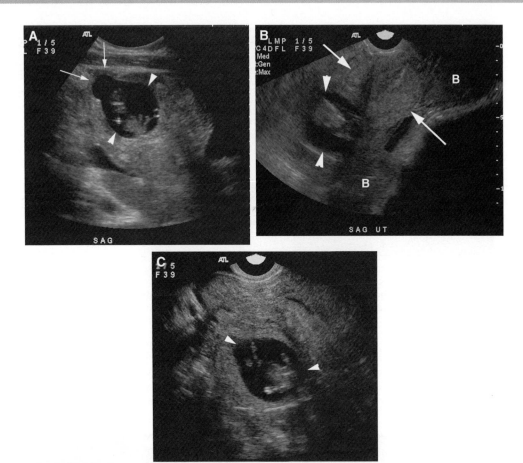

Fig. 12. Ruptured isthmic pregnancy at 11 weeks gestational age. (*A*) Sagittal transabdominal image shows a gestational sac (*arrowheads*) located high in the uterus, with the superior portion of the sac (*thin arrows*) bulging beyond the confines of the uterus. (*B,C*) Sagittal transvaginal images show blood (*B*) surrounding the uterus (*arrows*). The gestational sac (*arrowheads*) is again noted to be high in the uterus, without myometrium around the superior portion of the sac. At surgery a ruptured isthmic pregnancy was found.

sac or embryo is less commonly seen, with the appearance of the contents lagging in comparison with the gestational age. Abdominal pain before 7 weeks gestational age is typically present [81].

Abdominal pregnancies are rare. The pregnancy typically develops in the ligaments of the ovary, usually the broad ligament. It can then obtain blood supply from the omentum and abdominal organs. Sonographically, the pregnancy is seen separate from the uterus, adnexa, and ovaries. Treatment is by laparotomy or laparoscopy [82]. Abdominal pregnancy can result in a life-threatening emergency. However, if diagnosed late in gestation, a viable pregnancy can result.

Ovarian hyperstimulation

Ovarian hyperstimulation is diagnosed by the presence of abdominal pain, enlargement of the ovary greater than 5 cm, and ascites or hydrothorax

[83]. In addition, one of the following criteria has to be met: hematocrit 45% or more, white blood cells greater than 15,000/ml, oliguria, elevated liver enzymes, dyspnea, anasarca, or acute renal failure [83]. These patients may benefit by sonographically guided drainage of hyperstimulated ovaries to relieve the abdominal pain and distension they experience. One problem in the diagnosis of ovarian hyperstimulation is that if the patient is pregnant, ectopic pregnancy is still a possibility. If the pain is severe, torsion may also be present [Fig. 14].

Ovarian torsion

Ovarian torsion is the most frequent and most serious complication of benign ovarian cysts during pregnancy. Torsion is most common in the first trimester, and may result in cyst rupture into the peritoneal cavity. Symptoms include abdominal pain and tenderness that are usually sudden in onset,

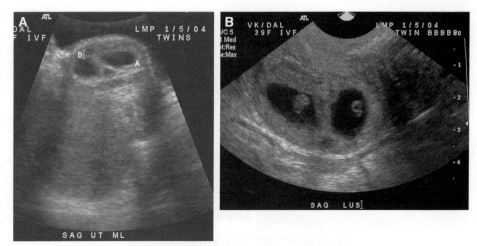

Fig. 13. Twin gestation in cesarean section scar. (*A*) Transabdominal view of a retroflexed uterus shows two gestational sacs (*A,B*) in the region of a prior cesarean section scar. (*B*) Transvaginal image shows embryos within the gestational sacs. These are in the anterior myometrium, separate from the endometrial cavity. The patient was given systemic methotrexate and the embryos were injected with potassium chloride.

and localized to the torsed ovary. Ultrasound frequently demonstrates an adnexal mass, and may show altered blood flow on Doppler studies. Doppler of ovarian torsion can be difficult because the ovaries have a dual blood supply, from the ovarian artery laterally and from the ovarian branch of the uterine artery medially. Presence of venous flow is predictive of ovarian viability [84]. In difficult cases, the authors have found MRI to be helpful in confirming the diagnosis of torsion [Fig. 15] [85].

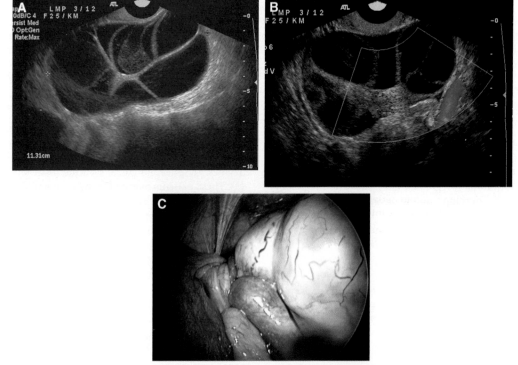

Fig. 14. Hyperstimulated torsed ovary in patient 7 weeks pregnant with severe pain. (*A*) Transverse sonogram demonstrates an enlarged left ovary measuring 11 cm with multiple cysts consistent with the patient's history of hyperstimulation. (*B*) Color Doppler shows flow in the ovary. Pulsed Doppler (not shown) demonstrated both arterial and venous flow. (*C*) Image at surgery shows torsion of the hyperstimulated ovary.

Fibroids

Uterine fibroids are commonly found during pregnancy. One in 500 pregnant women is admitted for a complication related to a fibroid [86]. Inconsistency of uterine size and gestational dates in a pregnant patient who has acute abdominal pain may be the first sign of leiomyoma. Fibroids during pregnancy occasionally undergo red degeneration that is caused by hemorrhagic infarction. The symptoms and signs are focal pain, with tenderness on palpation and sometimes low-grade fever. Moderate leukocytosis is common. The greatest increase in volume of myomas occurs before the 10th week of gestation. Fibroids either remain unchanged or increase in size in the first trimester as a response to increased estrogen [87]. The sonographic diagnosis of a degenerating fibroid is made when the patient experiences pain when the probe is placed over the fibroid. At times a lucent center will be visualized [Fig. 16].

Urinary tract

The urinary system undergoes many changes during pregnancy. The enlarging uterus puts pressure on the ureters, which can partially obstruct the normal downward flow of urine. Pregnancy also increases

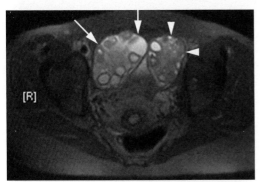

Fig. 15. Ovarian torsion in patient with twins after in vitro fertilization with severe intermittent right lower quadrant pain (11 weeks pregnant). Sonogram (not shown) had demonstrated enlarged ovaries with flow. Due to severe pain, an MR was performed. Axial fat saturated, T_2-weighted, single-shot, fast-spin echo image shows large ovaries, right (*arrows*) greater than left (*arrowheads*), with multiple follicles, consistent with history of hyperstimulation. The stroma of the right ovary is brighter than the left, consistent with edema caused by torsion. At surgery the ovary was edematous with 360° of torsion. (*From* Levine D, Pedrosa I. MR imaging of the maternal abdomen and pelvis in pregnancy. In: Levine D, editor. Atlas of fetal MRI. Boca Raton (FL): Taylor & Francis Group; 2005. p. 216; © 2005. Reproduced by permission of Routledge/Taylor & Francis Group, LLC.)

the risk of reflux of urine by causing the ureters to dilate and reducing the muscle contractions that propel urine downwards into the bladder. These changes make urinary tract infections very common. Many women who have bacteriuria will develop pyelonephritis during pregnancy. Both cystitis and pyelonephritis can be a cause of pelvic pain.

Although hydronephrosis of pregnancy can cause flank pain, is not a typical cause of pelvic pain. The appearance of dilated tracts can be confusing in pregnancy, however, because hydronephrosis can be caused by physiologic dilation of pregnancy, nephrolithiasis, or structural abnormalities.

Nephrolithiasis is an uncommon but important condition in pregnant women. The most common presenting complaint is flank pain.; however, when the stone is at the ureterovescicle junction, the patient may present with pelvic pain [Fig. 17]. The incidence of nephrolithiasis in pregnancy is about 1 per 2000 pregnancies [88]. If the ureter is dilated and a stone is not visualized, it can be helpful to assess for urinary jets in the bladder; however, these jets can be absent in cases without stones, and present with nonobstructing stones [89,90].

Gastrointestinal causes of pelvic pain

Acute appendicitis is the most common nonobstetrical surgical condition of the abdomen complicating pregnancy. Although the incidence of appendicitis occurring in pregnant women is considered to be the same as in nonpregnant women, the signs and symptoms and the laboratory findings usually associated with appendicitis in the nonpregnant condition are frequently unreliable during pregnancy [91]. On ultrasound, the abnormal

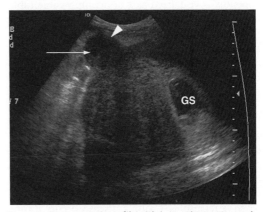

Fig. 16. Degenerating fibroid in patient 10 weeks pregnant. Transabdominal view of the uterus shows a gestational sac (*GS*) and an anterior fibroid (*arrowhead*) with a small lucency centrally (*thin arrow*). The patient was focally tender over the fibroid.

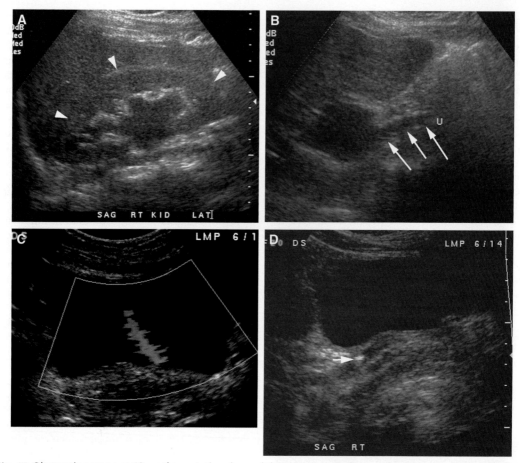

Fig. 17. Obstructing stone at 13 weeks gestational age. (*A*) Sagittal view of the right kidney (*arrowheads*) demonstrates hydronephrosis. (*B*) Sagittal view of the uteropelvic junction demonstrates dilation of the proximal right ureter (*U, long arrows*). (*C*) Transverse view of the bladder with color shows a left ureteral jet but no right jet was demonstrated. (*D*) View of the right ureterovescicle junction demonstrates a small stone (*small arrow*) without a shadow.

appendix is visualized as a noncompressible tubular structure measuring 6 mm or greater in the region of the patient's pain [Fig. 18]. An appendicolith or periappendiceal fluid may be visualized. If ultrasound diagnosis is inadequate, MRI can be helpful in assessing the etiology of right-sided pain in pregnancy [92,93].

Crohn's disease can also be a cause of pelvic pain in pregnancy. Most pregnant women who have a history of inflammatory bowel disease have uneventful pregnancies, and exacerbations of disease can be controlled with medical therapy. Although it is rare for the new onset of inflammatory bowel disease to be diagnosed during pregnancy [94], when a relapse of Crohn's disease occurs during pregnancy, it typically will occur during the first trimester [95]. Imaging can start with ultrasound, but frequently another modality is needed, such as MRI or CT.

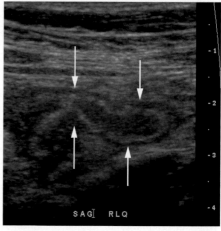

Fig. 18. Appendicitis in pregnancy. Oblique view in the right lower quadrant demonstrates the dilated appendix (*arrows*).

Summary

Pelvic pain during the first trimester of pregnancy can pose a challenge to the clinician. Ultrasound is a very important imaging modality in evaluating these patients.

References

[1] Chiang G, Levine D, Swire M, et al. The intradecidual sign: is it reliable for diagnosis of early intrauterine pregnancy? AJR Am J Roentgenol 2004;183:725–31.

[2] Yeh HC. Efficacy of the intradecidual sign and fallacy of the double decidual sac sign in the diagnosis of early intrauterine pregnancy. Radiology 1999;210:579–82.

[3] Yeh HC, Goodman JD, Carr L, et al. Intradecidual sign: a US criterion of early intrauterine pregnancy. Radiology 1986;161:463–7.

[4] Bradley WG, Fiske CE, Filly RA. The double sac sign of early intrauterine pregnancy: use in exclusion of ectopic pregnancy. Radiology 1982;143:223–6.

[5] Levi CS, Lyons EA, Lindsay DJ. Ultrasound in the first trimester of pregnancy. Radiol Clin North Am 1990;28:19–38.

[6] Levi CS, Lyons EA, Zheng XH, et al. Endovaginal US: demonstration of cardiac activity in embryos of less than 5.0 mm in crown-rump length. Radiology 1990;176:71–4.

[7] Pearlstone M, Baxi L. Subchorionic hematoma: a review. Obstet Gynecol Surv 1993;48:65–8.

[8] Mantoni M, Pedersen JF. Intrauterine haematoma. An ultrasonic study of threatened abortion. Br J Obstet Gynaecol 1981;88:47–51.

[9] Ball RH, Ade CM, Schoenborn JA, et al. The clinical significance of ultransonographically detected subchorionic hemorrhages. Am J Obstet Gynecol 1996;174:996–1002.

[10] Nagy S, Bush M, Stone J, et al. Clinical significance of subchorionic and retroplacental hematomas detected in the first trimester of pregnancy. Obstet Gynecol 2003;102:94–100.

[11] Simpson J, Carson S. Genetic and non-genetic casues of spontaneous abortions. In: Sciarra J, editor. Gynecology and obstetrics. Philadelphia: JB Lippencott; 1995. p. 20.

[12] Filly RA. Ultrasound evaluation during the first trimester. In: Callen PW, editor. Ultrasonography in obstetrics and gynecology. Philadelphia: WB Saunders; 1998. p. 63–85.

[13] McKenna KM, Feldstein VA, Goldstein RB, et al. The empty amnion: a sign of early pregnancy failure. J Ultrasound Med 1995;14:117–21.

[14] Szulman AE, Surti U. The syndromes of hydatidiform mole. II. Morphologic evolution of the complete and partial mole. Am J Obstet Gynecol 1978;132:20–7.

[15] Lazarus E, Hulka C, Siewert B, et al. Sonographic appearance of early complete molar pregnancies. J Ultrasound Med 1999;18:589–94.

[16] Chiang G, Levine D. Imaging of adnexal masses in pregnancy. J Ultrasound Med 2004;23:805–19.

[17] Patel MD, Feldstein VA, Filly RA. The likelihood ratio of sonographic findings for the diagnosis of hemorrhagic ovarian cysts. J Ultrasound Med 2005;24:607–15.

[18] Jain KA. Sonographic spectrum of hemorrhagic ovarian cysts. J Ultrasound Med 2002;21:879–86.

[19] Russell SA, Filly RA, Damato N. Sonographic diagnosis of ectopic pregnancy with endovaginal probes: what really has changed? J Ultrasound Med 1993;12:145–51.

[20] Nyberg DA, Hughes MP, Mack LA, et al. Extrauterine findings of ectopic pregnancy of transvaginal US: importance of echogenic fluid. Radiology 1991;178:823–6.

[21] Aboud E. A five-year review of ectopic pregnancy. Clin Exp Obstet Gynecol 1997;24:127–9.

[22] From the Centers for Disease Control and Prevention. Ectopic pregnancy—United States, 1990–1992. JAMA 1995;273:533.

[23] Chow WH, Daling JR, Cates W Jr, et al. Epidemiology of ectopic pregnancy. Epidemiol Rev 1987;9:70–94.

[24] DeVoe RW, Pratt JH. Simultaneous intra- and extrauterine pregnancy. Am J Obstet Gynecol 1948;56:1119.

[25] Richards SR, Stempel LE, Carlton BD. Heterotopic pregnancy: reappraisal of incidence. Am J Obstet Gynecol 1982;142:928–30.

[26] Bello GV, Schonholz D, Moshirpur J, et al. Combined pregnancy: the Mount Sinai experience. Obstet Gynecol Surv 1986;41:603–13.

[27] Berger MJ, Taymor ML. Simultaneous intrauterine and tubal pregnancies following ovulation induction. Am J Obstet Gynecol 1972;113:812–3.

[28] Cacciatore B, Ulf-hakan S, Ylostalo P. Diagnosis of ectopic pregnancy by vaginal ultrasonography in combination with a discriminatory serum hCG level of 1000 IU/l (IRP). Br J Obstet Gynaecol 1990;97:904–8.

[29] Barnhart K, Mennuti MT, Benjamin I, et al. Prompt diagnosis of ectopic pregnancy in an emergency department setting. Obstet Gynecol 1994;84:1010–5.

[30] Mehta TS, Levine D, Beckwith B. Treatment of ectopic pregnancy: is a human chorionic gonadotropin level of 2,000 mIU/mL a reasonable threshold? Radiology 1997;205:569–73.

[31] Bateman BG, Nunley WC, Kolp LA, et al. Vaginal sonography findings and hCG dynamics of early intrauterine and tubal pregnancies. Obstet Gynecol 1990;75:421–7.

[32] Goldstein SR, Snyder JR, Watson C, et al. Very early pregnancy detection with endovaginal ultrasound. Obstet Gynecol 1988;72:200–4.

[33] Sauer MV, Gorrill MJ, Rodi IA, et al. Nonsurgical management of unruptured ectopic pregnancy: an extended clinical trial. Fertil Steril 1987;48:752–5.

[34] Fernandez H, Rainhorn JD, Papiernik E, et al. Spontaneous resolution of ectopic pregnancy. Obstet Gynecol 1988;71:171–4.

[35] Atri M, Bret PM, Tulandi T. Spontaneous resolution of ectopic pregnancy: initial appearance and evolution at transvaginal US. Radiology 1993; 186:83–6.

[36] Batzer R. Guidelines for choosing a pregnancy test. Contemp Ob Gyn 1985;30:57.

[37] Breen JL. A 21 year survey of 654 ectopic pregnancies. Am J Obstet Gynecol 1970;106: 1004–19.

[38] Dialani V, Levine D. Ectopic pregnancy: a review. Ultrasound Q 2004;20:105–17.

[39] Ackerman TE, Levi CS, Dashefsky SM, et al. Interstitial line: sonographic finding in interstitial (cornual) ectopic pregnancy. Radiology 1993; 189:83–7.

[40] Yeh HC. Some misconceptions and pitfalls in ultrasonography. Ultrasound Q 2001;17:129–55.

[41] Frates MC, Laing FC. Sonographic evaluation of ectopic pregnancy: an update. AJR Am J Roentgenol 1995;165:251–9.

[42] Nyberg DA, Mack LA, Jeffrey RB Jr, et al. Endovaginal sonographic evaluation of ectopic pregnancy: a prospective study. AJR Am J Roentgenol 1987;149:1181–6.

[43] Atri M, de Stempel J, Bret PM. Accuracy of transvaginal ultrasonography for detection of hematosalpinx in ectopic pregnancy. J Clin Ultrasound 1992;20:255–61.

[44] Fleischer AC, Pennell RG, McKee MS, et al. Ectopic pregnancy: features at transvaginal sonography. Radiology 1990;174:375–8.

[45] Cacciatore B. Can the status of tubal pregnancy be predicted with transvaginal sonography? A prospective comparison of sonographic, surgical, and serum hCG findings. Radiology 1990;177: 481–4.

[46] Nyberg DA, Mack LA, Laing FC, et al. Early pregnancy complications: endovaginal sonographic findings correlated with human chorionic gonadotropin levels. Radiology 1988; 167:619–22.

[47] Cacciatore B, Stenman UH, Ylostalo P. Early screening for ectopic pregnancy in high-risk symptom-free women. Lancet 1994;343:517–8.

[48] Cacciatore B, Stenman U-H, Ylostalo P. Comparison of abdominal and vaginal sonography in suspected ectopic pregnancy. Obstet Gynecol 1989;73:770–4.

[49] Dashefsky SM, Lyons EA, Levi CS, et al. Suspected ectopic pregnancy: endovaginal and transvesical US. Radiology 1988;169:181–4.

[50] Thorsen MK, Lawson TL, Aiman EJ, et al. Diagnosis of ectopic pregnancy: endovaginal vs transabdominal sonography. AJR Am J Roentgenol 1990;155:307–10.

[51] Kivikoski AI, Martin CM, Smeltzer JS. Transabdominal and transvaginal ultrasonography in the diagnosis of ectopic pregnancy: a comparative study. Am J Obstet Gynecol 1990;163:123–8.

[52] Frates MC, Brown DL, Doubilet PM, et al. Tubal rupture in patients with ectopic pregnancy: diagnosis with transvaginal US. Radiology 1994;191: 769–72.

[53] Brown DL, Doubilet PM. Transvaginal sonography for diagnosing ectopic pregnancy: positivity criteria and performance characteristics. J Ultrasound Med 1994;13:259–66.

[54] Stiller RJ, Haynes de Regt R, Blair E. Transvaginal ultrasonography in patients at risk for ectopic pregnancy. Am J Obstet Gynecol 1989;161: 930–3.

[55] Filly RA. Ectopic pregnancy: the role of sonography. Radiology 1987;162:661–8.

[56] Frates MC, Visweswaran A, Laing FC. Comparison of tubal ring and corpus luteum echogenicities: a useful differentiating characteristic. J Ultrasound Med 2001;20:27–31.

[57] Stein MW, Ricci ZJ, Novak L, et al. Sonographic comparison of the tubal ring of ectopic pregnancy with the corpus luteum. J Ultrasound Med 2004;23:57–62.

[58] Emerson DS, Cartier MS, Altieri LA, et al. Diagnostic efficacy of endovaginal color Doppler flow imaging in an ectopic pregnancy screening program. Radiology 1992;183:413–20.

[59] Levine D. Ectopic pregnancy. In: Callen PW, editor. Ultrasonography in obstetrics and gynecology. Pennsylvania: WB Saunders Co.; 2000. p. 912–34.

[60] Swire MN, Castro-Aragon I, Levine D. Various sonographic appearances of the hemorrhagic corpus luteum cyst. Ultrasound Q 2004;20: 45–58.

[61] Taylor KJ, Meyer WR. New techniques in the diagnosis of ectopic pregnancy. Obstet Gynecol Clin North Am 1991;18:39–54.

[62] Bouyer J, Coste J, Fernandez H, et al. Sites of ectopic pregnancy: a 10 year population-based study of 1800 cases. Hum Reprod 2002;17: 3224–30.

[63] Jafri SZ, Loginsky SJ, Bouffard JA, et al. Sonographic detection of interstitial pregnancy. J Clin Ultrasound 1987;15:253–7.

[64] Lee GS, Hur SY, Kown I, et al. Diagnosis of early intramural ectopic pregnancy. J Clin Ultrasound 2005;33:190–2.

[65] Chen GD, Lin MT, Lee MS. Diagnosis of interstitial pregnancy with sonography. J Clin Ultrasound 1994;22:439–42.

[66] Fernandez H, Benifla JL, Lelaidier C, et al. Methotrexate treatment of ectopic pregnancy: 100 cases treated by primary transvaginal injection under sonographic control. Fertil Steril 1993; 59:773–7.

[67] Doubilet PM, Benson CB, Frates MC, et al. Sonographically guided minimally invasive treatment of unusual ectopic pregnancies. J Ultrasound Med 2004;23:359–70.

[68] Celik C, Bala A, Acar A, et al. Methotrexate for cervical pregnancy. A case report. J Reprod Med 2003;48:130–2.

[69] Ushakov FB, Elchalal U, Aceman PJ, et al. Cervical pregnancy: past and future. Obstet Gynecol Surv 1997;52:45–59.

[70] Monteagudo A, Tarricone NJ, Timor-Tritsch IE, et al. Successful transvaginal ultrasound-guided puncture and injection of a cervical pregnancy in a patient with simultaneous intrauterine pregnancy and a history of a previous cervical pregnancy. Ultrasound Obstet Gynecol 1996;8: 381–6.

[71] Frates MC, Benson CB, Doubilet PM, et al. Cervical ectopic pregnancy: results of conservative treatment. Radiology 1994;191:773–5.

[72] Jurkovic D, Hacket E, Campbell S. Diagnosis and treatment of early cervical pregnancy: a review and a report of two cases treated conservatively. Ultrasound Obstet Gynecol 1996;8: 373–80.

[73] Stovall TG, Ling FW. Ectopic pregnancy. Diagnostic and therapeutic algorithms minimizing surgical intervention. J Reprod Med 1993;38: 807–12.

[74] Sherer DM, Abramowicz JS, Thompson HO, et al. Comparison of transabdominal and endovaginal sonographic approaches in the diagnosis of a case of cervical pregnancy successfully treated with methotrexate. J Ultrasound Med 1991;10:409–11.

[75] Meyerovitz MF, Lobel SM, Harrington DP, et al. Preoperative uterine artery embolization in cervical pregnancy. J Vasc Interv Radiol 1991;2: 95–7.

[76] Jurkovic D, Hillaby K, Woelfer B, et al. First-trimester diagnosis and management of pregnancies implanted into the lower uterine segment Cesarean section scar. Ultrasound Obstet Gynecol 2003;21:220–7.

[77] Li SP, Wang W, Tang XL, et al. Cesarean scar pregnancy: a case report. Chin Med J (Engl) 2004; 117:316–7.

[78] Seow KM, Huang LW, Lin YH, et al. Cesarean scar pregnancy: issues in management. Ultrasound Obstet Gynecol 2004;23:247–53.

[79] Haimov-Kochman R, Sciaky-Tamir Y, Yanai N, et al. Conservative management of two ectopic pregnancies implanted in previous uterine scars. Ultrasound Obstet Gynecol 2002;19:616–9.

[80] Fylstra DL. Ectopic pregnancy within a cesarean scar: a review. Obstet Gynecol Surv 2002;57: 537–43.

[81] Comstock C, Huston K, Lee W. The ultrasonographic appearance of ovarian ectopic pregnancies. Obstet Gynecol 2005;105:42–5.

[82] Siow A, Chern B, Soong Y. Successful laparoscopic treatment of an abdominal pregnancy in the broad ligament. Singapore Med J 2004;45:88–9.

[83] Practice Committee of the American Society of Reproductive Medicine. Ovarian hyperstimulation syndrome. Fertil Steril 2004;82(Suppl 1): S81–6.

[84] Fleischer AC, Stein SM, Cullinan JA, et al. Color Doppler sonography of adnexal torsion. J Ultrasound Med 1995;14:523–8.

[85] Levine D, Pedrosa I. MR imaging of the maternal abdomen and pelvis in pregnancy. In: Levine D, editor. Atlas of fetal MRI. Boca Raton (FL): Taylor & Francis Group; 2005. p. 175–92.

[86] Katz VL, Dotters DJ, Droegemeuller W. Complications of uterine leiomyomas in pregnancy. Obstet Gynecol 1989;73:593–6.

[87] Lev-Toaff AS, Coleman BG, Arger PH, et al. Leiomyomas in pregnancy: sonographic study. Radiology 1987;164:375–80.

[88] Hendricks SK, Ross SO, Krieger JN. An algorithm for diagnosis and therapy of management and complications of urolithiasis during pregnancy. Surg Gynecol Obstet 1991;172:49–54.

[89] Deyoe LA, Cronan JJ, Breslaw BH, et al. New techniques of ultrasound and color Doppler in the prospective evaluation of acute renal obstruction. Do they replace the intravenous urogram? Abdom Imaging 1995;20:58–63.

[90] Geavlete P, Georgescu D, Cauni V, et al. Value of duplex Doppler ultrasonography in renal colic. Eur Urol 2002;41:71–8.

[91] Tamir IL, Bongard FS, Klein SR. Acute appendicitis in the pregnant patient. Am J Surg 1990;160: 571–5 [discussion: 575–6].

[92] Eyvazzadeh AD, Pedrosa I, Rofsky NM, et al. MRI of right-sided abdominal pain in pregnancy. AJR Am J Roentgenol 2004;183:907–14.

[93] Pedrosa I, Levine D, Eyvazzadeh AD, et al. MRI evaluation of suspected acute appendicitis in pregnancy. Radiology, in press.

[94] Goettler CE, Stellato TA. Initial presentation of Crohn's disease in pregnancy: report of a case. Dis Colon Rectum 2003;46:406–10.

[95] Hill J, Clark A, Scott NA. Surgical treatment of acute manifestations of Crohn's disease during pregnancy. J R Soc Med 1997;90:64–6.

RADIOLOGIC
CLINICS
OF NORTH AMERICA

Radiol Clin N Am 44 (2006) 879–899

ELSEVIER
SAUNDERS

Practical Approach to the Adnexal Mass

Maitray D. Patel, MD

- Normal anatomy
- Overview of ultrasound analytic approach to the adnexal mass
- Unilocular smooth-walled anechoic cyst
- Physiologic causes of findings that may raise concern
- When physiologic process is unlikely, has a characteristic pattern been established?
  - *Non-neoplastic cyst*
  - *Endometrioma*

- *Hydrosalpinx*
- *Peritoneal inclusion cyst*
- *Cystic teratoma*
- *Benign and malignant cystic neoplasms (cystadenomas and cystadenocarcinomas)*
- *Other potentially characteristic adnexal masses*
- *Further imaging or surgical exploration*
- Summary
- References

Evaluation of an adnexal mass, either presenting on physical examination, suspected based on clinical history, or identified on routine pelvic sonography, is a common task for the sonologist. While the clinical context is very important, for the vast majority of sonographically identified adnexal masses, the subsequent management of the patient will be highly dependent on the sonologist's interpretation of the imaging findings. The sonologist who merely measures the size of a mass and who subsequently offers a differential diagnosis that includes nearly every adnexal abnormality, including malignancy, has failed in his or her opportunity to contribute meaningfully to the care of the patient. Using a practical approach [Fig. 1] and with knowledge of the sonographic patterns of adnexal pathology, the sonologist is better equipped to make reasoned conclusions and useful recommendations for patient management.

Normal anatomy

An understanding of the expected sonographic appearance of the ovary is important so that one does not confuse normal structures with pathology. The ovary is highly dynamic, with constant formation and regression of "physiologic cysts" even before menarche. During the menstrual cycle, hormonally mediated ovulation begins with the recruitment of about five to eight preantral follicles, which are visible as small cysts during the early proliferative phase measuring about 2 to 4 mm in diameter [1]. A dominant follicle emerges by days 8 to 10 of the cycle, generally measuring about 10 mm in diameter, exceeding the diameter of the other follicles. Occasionally two dominant follicles will develop, but not in the same ovary [2]. Both dominant and nondominant follicles increase in size until ovulation; the dominant follicle is

This article was originally published in *Ultrasound Clinics* 1:2, April 2006.
Department of Radiology, Mayo Clinic, 13400 E. Shea Blvd., Scottsdale, AZ 85259, USA
E-mail address: patel.maitray@mayo.edu

doi:10.1016/j.rcl.2006.10.016

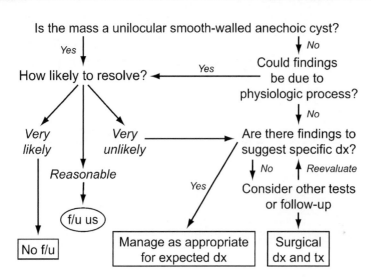

Fig. 1. Suggested approach to the sonographically identified adnexal mass.

expected to become 2 to 2.5 cm in average diameter. In contrast, nondominant follicles typically do not exceed 1.1 cm in size [Fig. 2] [3].

With ovulation, the dominant follicle ruptures, typically losing much if not all of its internal fluid and collapsing into a sonographically "solid" appearing structure (if visible at all). This becomes the corpus luteum; the margins of the corpus luteum are hypervascular, leading to a "ring of fire" appearance on color Doppler sonography, and they may be thick and somewhat irregular, reflecting the loss of wall tension following rupture [Fig. 3] [4]. The corpus luteum is typically smaller than the mature follicle from which it arose, measuring about 1.5 cm. Hemorrhage into the corpus luteum can lead to re-expansion, resulting in a hemorrhagic ovarian cyst [Fig. 4]; the size of the cyst varies, but it is not unusual for it to be up to 4 cm in diameter.

Recognizing this normal physiologic process is paramount to avoiding the temptation to view every ovarian cyst as a mass requiring treatment or follow-up imaging. Some experts have advocated that sonologists avoid using the term "cyst" to describe anything in the ovary which is likely to be secondary to normal physiologic events [5]. Certainly, use of the terms "follicle," "dominant follicle," and "corpus luteum" in sonographic reports serves to describe these structures without inadvertently misleading others to believe that they are findings that are potentially pathologic. With even just a little experience, and with some attention to the phase of the menstrual cycle at which time the premenopausal patient is being imaged, sonologists should have no difficulty in ignoring these expected normal ovarian findings when they appear typical, as they will in the vast majority of cases.

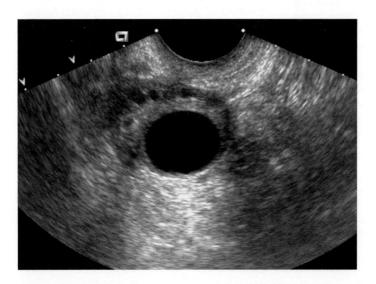

Fig. 2. Dominant follicle. Sonogram of an ovary in a premenopausal woman shows a unilocular smooth-walled anechoic cyst measuring 2.5 cm in maximum diameter, with multiple other follicles in the ovarian parenchyma. This is the expected appearance of a dominant follicle in a premenopausal woman.

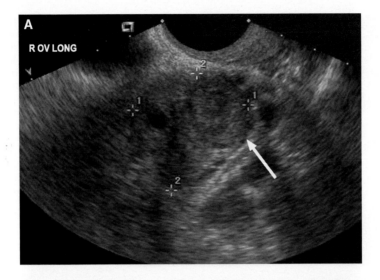

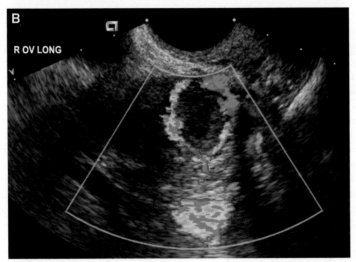

Fig. 3. Corpus Luteum. (*A*) Sonogram of an ovary (demarcated by electonic calipers) in a premenopausal woman shows the corpus luteum (*arrow*) as a predominantly solid-appearing structure within the ovarian parenchyma, with a thick wall and internal echoes. (*B*) The rim of the corpus luteum shows hypervascularity as compared with the rest of the ovary, resulting in an appearance on color Doppler sonography that has been called a "ring-of-fire."

Nevertheless, some of these physiologic structures will develop into larger masses or exhibit atypical features requiring an analytic approach by the so-nologist for further evaluation.

Overview of ultrasound analytic approach to the adnexal mass

The sonographer who uses a practical approach to imaging recognizes that there are specific categories or groupings of pathologic processes that can result in an adnexal mass. The approach seeks to deter-mine if a sonographically identified mass exhibits an imaging pattern that is reasonably characteristic of a particular category. Some categories are broad, encompassing several different pathologic entities, whereas others are more specific, referring to a single pathologic entity; as a result, the categories overlap for some entities. The categories with potentially characteristic imaging features are as follows, listed in a morphologic spectrum from unilocular and entirely cystic to variable/multilocular/partially cystic to entirely solid: (1) non-neoplastic cyst; (2) hemorrhagic ovarian cyst; (3) endometrioma; (4) hydrosalpinx; (5) perito-neal inclusion cyst; (6) benign cystic neoplasm; (7) cystic teratoma; (8) cystic malignancy; (9) ec-topic pregnancy; (10) abscess/inflammatory mass;

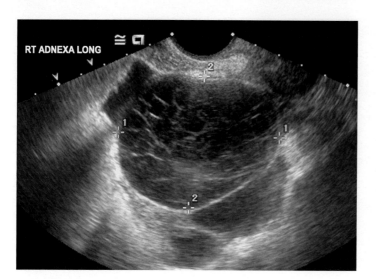

Fig. 4. Hemorrhagic ovarian cyst. Sonogram of an ovary in a premenopausal woman shows a cyst (demarcated by electronic calipers) measuring over 6 cm in diameter, containing multiple internal fibrin strands. These characteristic fibrin strands should not be misinterpreted as septations.

(11) torsed ovary; (12) exophytic or broad ligament myoma; (13) ovarian fibroma; and (14) solid mass.

At the most basic level, the sonologist's approach to the sonographically identified adnexal mass can be understood as a two-phase process. First, the sonologist determines if the mass exhibits a characteristic pattern indicating the likely cause or category. If so, the mass is managed as appropriate for that type of pathology in the clinical context of the patient. If not, the sonologist considers if a subsequent diagnostic test (including repeat follow-up ultrasound) can be used to safely allow potential characterization of the mass into a particular pathologic category and thereby avoid surgery or improve surgical planning. If so, the subsequent test or follow-up should be recommended. If not, diagnostic surgical evaluation will be indicated. In essence, the imager confronting an adnexal mass asks two questions: do I know what this is with reasonable certainty? If not, is there a test or strategy that has a reasonable chance of enabling me to know what this is and that would make a difference in the care of the patient?

Note the emphasis on pattern recognition in this approach; it all boils down to whether one can be reasonably certain of the pathology. Research indicates that subjective evaluation of ovarian masses using pattern recognition achieves high sensitivity and specificity for discriminating malignant pathology from benign pathology [6,7]. Furthermore, investigations have quantified a high likelihood ratio for specific sets of observations that enable sonologists to confidently discriminate particular causes of adnexal pathology [8–11]. When specific sonographic observations and considerations are placed in the framework of the basic practical approach (do I know what this is? if not, is there a test or strategy that will enable me to know

what this is and make a difference to the care of the patient?), the sonologist is able to render effective recommendations for the management of the identified adnexal mass.

Fig. 1 details a specific algorithm that expands on this basic practical approach by detailing a step-by-step analysis that facilitates understanding what a mass is likely to be and what should be done next. The critical questions to be answered are: (1) is the mass a unilocular anechoic smooth-walled cyst?; if so, how likely is it to be a non-neoplastic cyst that will not require treatment?; (2) if the mass is not a cyst that is unilocular, anechoic, and smooth-walled, is it possible that normal physiologic changes might account for the aberrant observations?; if so, how likely is the mass to be a non-neoplastic cyst that will not require treatment?; (3) if normal physiologic changes do not likely explain the aberrant observations, can one identify other observations that enable classification into a particular category?; (4) if sonographic observations are insufficient to allow characterization as a particular pathologic category, are there other diagnostic tests that could be used that might reasonably assist in placing the mass in a single category?; if so, would that be clinically meaningful?

The remainder of this article focuses on detailing the sonographic observations and considerations relevant to the questions posed by the algorithm, with primary attention to those masses with cystic features. The adnexal mass related to ectopic pregnancy or inflammation/abscess almost always arises in a specific clinical setting that has unique analytic considerations separate from the focus of this discussion, and these entities will not be further discussed. Likewise, there is no discussion regarding the sonographic patterns of ovarian torsion and various categories of adnexal solid masses. The recommended imaging algorithm for an adnexal mass can and should be applied to these entities, but discussion of the analysis of these masses is beyond the scope of this article.

Unilocular smooth-walled anechoic cyst

The first step in analysis of the sonographically identified adnexal mass is to decide if it meets the criteria for a unilocular anechoic smooth-walled cyst. These cysts are common in premenopausal women, since essentially every nonhemorrhagic dominant follicle could be thus described. With the increasing use of ultrasound, it has been firmly established over the last few decades that these cysts are also common in postmenopausal women. The incidence of such cysts in postmenopausal women has been reported to be up to 20% [12–14]. These cysts are round or oval in shape, have no internal structure or echogenicity, and have a clearly demonstrable wall without defined surface projections or nodularity [Fig. 5]. A cyst with slight crenulation of the wall resulting in mild irregularity would still be considered smooth-walled if no clearly defined surface projections are evident.

There are practically two pathologic possibilities when a unilocular anechoic smooth-walled adnexal cyst is identified: either the mass is a non-neoplastic cyst or it is a benign cystic neoplasm. The term "non-neoplastic cyst" is a very useful imaging designation but not highly specific. A number of specific pathologic entities can fall into this category, including physiologic cysts (cysts that develop in the course of ovulation, namely the follicular cyst and corpus luteum cyst), theca lutein cysts, serous inclusion cysts, endometriomas, peritoneal inclusion cysts, and paraovarian/paratubal cysts. Some of these pathologic entities may demonstrate other sonographic features that enable more specific categorization; for example, sonographic identification of a separate ovary will allow more specific categorization of a unilocular smooth-walled anechoic cyst as a paraovarian cyst. Furthermore, not every individual pathologic entity in this list will always appear as a unilocular anechoic smooth-walled cyst; for example, the vast majority of endometriomas will contain low-level echoes [8].

It is important to have confidence in the fact that the risk of malignancy is extremely low when a mass is assuredly characterized as a unilocular smooth-walled cyst. The data supporting this conclusion are extensive. Based on the natural history of more than 3000 unilocular ovarian cysts identified in postmenopausal women measuring 10 cm or less in diameter, Modesitt and colleagues [13] calculate a risk of malignancy of less than 0.1% with 95% confidence interval. The rare unilocular smooth-walled cyst that does eventually prove to be malignant (usually borderline) has papillary projections or septations identified on follow-up [13]. These rare malignancies may be misclassified as unilocular smooth-walled cysts on initial evaluation by failure to identify the wall nodularity [15]. Size is also an important consideration; the rare borderline tumor or malignancy that appears to be a unilocular anechoic smooth-walled cyst is nearly always over 5 cm in diameter [15].

Distinguishing between a non-neoplastic cyst and a benign neoplasm is clinically relevant. Non-neoplastic cysts are often self-limiting and resolve without intervention. The main risk of an asymptomatic non-neoplastic ovarian cyst that does not resolve spontaneously is that it can theoretically induce torsion of the ovary, though the risk of this event must be very low, given the commonality of non-neoplastic cysts and the infrequency of torsion.

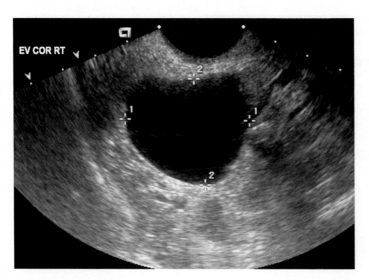

Fig. 5. Unilocular smooth-walled anechoic cyst. Sonogram of the right ovary in this postmenopausal patient shows a cyst meeting criteria for designation as a unilocular smooth-walled anechoic cyst. In this case, the cyst measures just over 3.5 cm in maximum diameter. Minimal irregularity at the 5 o'clock position of the cyst is not sufficient to raise concern.

Thus, if one can be reasonably confident that an adnexal mass is due to a non-neoplastic cyst, there are several management options. One could choose to ignore the mass as long as the patient remained asymptomatic, assuming that it will disappear over time. Alternatively, one could elect to percutaneously aspirate and treat the cyst [Fig. 6] [16]; this course of action is less frequently chosen, usually only for those non-neoplastic cysts that are of certain size and that have not resolved over time. Indications for this maneuver might include localized patient discomfort related to the volume of the mass and its effect on adjacent organs, such as the urinary bladder. Of course, surgical management remains an option if the patient is symptomatic or desires removal.

On the other hand, a unilocular smooth-walled cyst that has a reasonable chance of being a benign neoplasm is almost always surgically removed. First, there is a concern about the rare malignancy appearing to be a unilocular smooth-walled cyst. Even if one could be further assured of the benignity of a mass by evaluation of CA-125 levels or other considerations [17], benign neglect of a mass which has features suggesting a benign neoplasm rather than a non-neoplastic cyst is not a long-term option as it can be expected to lead only to a situation that will have to be addressed later, either emergently if the mass induces ovarian torsion or electively as the mass enlarges and causes symptoms. Percutaneous drainage of a cystic mass likely to be a benign neoplasm rather than a non-neoplastic cyst could also be considered, but this approach remains controversial [16].

There are four factors to consider when trying to distinguish between a non-neoplastic cyst and a benign neoplasm as the cause of a unilocular anechoic smooth-walled mass: location, growth rate, menopausal status, and size. Location is the most obvious consideration, as identification of a clearly separate ovary nearly eliminates the possibility of a benign neoplasm [Fig. 7]. There are exceptions to every rule, and in this regard, there are reports of paraovarian cystadenomas [18,19]; nevertheless, for practical purposes one can reasonably designate a mass as very likely being a non-neoplastic cyst when a clearly separate ipsilateral ovary is identified.

Consideration of the growth rate of the cyst can also be fruitful in distinguishing between a non-neoplastic cyst and a benign neoplasm. Cysts that can be documented to have appeared suddenly, always in premenopausal women, are clearly non-neoplastic physiologic cysts. Thus, a patient who had a sonogram within the preceding few months demonstrating normal ovaries without mass, who then returns for evaluation of rapid onset of unilateral adnexal pain wherein a 4 cm ovarian cyst is identified, clearly has a non-neoplastic cyst as the cause of the mass. Neoplasms do not exhibit this type of "hypergrowth." Similarly, cysts that are shown to have long-term stability are undoubtedly non-neoplastic (however, a pathologist may designate such a cyst as a cystadenoma if it eventually gets surgically removed, because the pathologic distinction between a cystadenoma and some types of non-neoplastic ovarian cysts can be imprecise). Finally, any cyst that demonstrates reduction in size is clearly not neoplastic.

Size and hormonal status are important considerations when a unilocular smooth-walled cyst is encountered, not only to suggest whether the cyst is non-neoplastic or a benign neoplasm but also determine the intensity of additional testing to

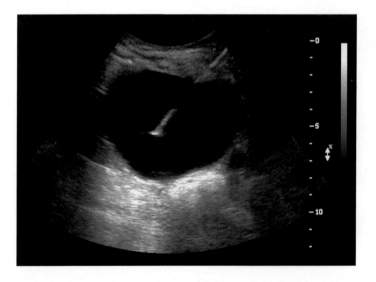

Fig. 6. Percutaneous aspiration of a unilocular smooth-walled anechoic cyst. Sonogram of a persistent left adnexal cyst in a perimenopausal woman documents the percutaneous insertion of a needle. The cyst was completely aspirated. In this case, the cyst had been demonstrated to be 50% larger on a prior sonogram 18 months ago. It was stable since the previous sonogram 6 months ago.

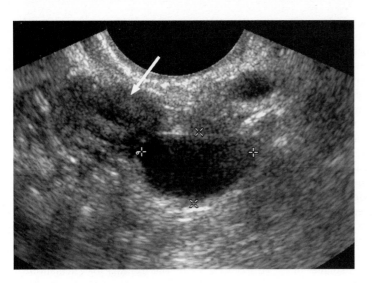

Fig. 7. Paraovarian cyst. Sonogram of the left adnexa in an asymptomatic postmenopausal woman shows a unilocular smooth-walled anechoic cyst (demarcated with electronic calipers). An adjacent normal appearing ovary is also identified (*arrow*). Other images (not shown) confirmed the impression that the cyst was abutting but not arising from the ovary. Follow-up sonograms were not requested as long as the patient remained asymptomatic.

recommend. Keeping in mind that normal physiologic events are expected to result in the development of a dominant follicle and a corpus luteum in every normal ovulatory cycle in a premenopausal woman, unilocular smooth-walled cysts below a certain size in premenopausal women can be assumed to be non-neoplastic in the absence of contrary clinical features. There is no magic number below which benign neoplasm becomes theoretically impossible; likewise, there is no magic number above which non-neoplastic cyst is theoretically excluded. A practical approach that I use is to consider a unilocular smooth-walled anechoic cyst in a premenopausal or perimenopausal woman measuring 4 cm or less in average diameter as very likely non-neoplastic in cause (I use the 4-cm threshold as a reasonable approach; some would use 3 cm, even if the woman is premenopausal). Conversely, a similar cyst in the same patient measuring 8 cm or larger is very likely a benign neoplasm. For postmenopausal women, I reduce the threshold by 3 cm; thus, a unilocular smooth-walled cyst measuring less than 1 cm in diameter is very likely non-neoplastic, and a similar cyst measuring over 5 cm is very likely a benign neoplasm. Those cysts that fall between these ranges are considered to be either a non-neoplastic cyst or benign neoplasm (distinction not yet possible). The probabilities favor non-neoplastic cyst at the lower end of the size range and benign neoplasm at the higher end of the size range, but additional testing (sonographic follow-up) would be appropriate.

Many sonographically identified unilocular smooth-walled cysts can be ignored; many do not require sonographic follow-up or surgical intervention. In fact, imagers who routinely recommend sonographic follow-up for a cyst that already exhibits features or behavior that indicates that it can be reasonably expected to be non-neoplastic force sonographic overuse. When a mass is very likely to be a non-neoplastic cyst, the imaging report might be worded as follows: "In the absence of persistent symptoms or other clinical considerations, sonographic follow-up should not be necessary." For example, this would be appropriate for the unilocular smooth-walled cyst measuring less than 4 cm in maximum size in a premenopausal woman, less than 1 cm in size in the post-menopausal woman, any cyst showing long-term stability, and any paraovarian unilocular smooth-walled cyst. (Some would opt to follow these cysts, likely non-neoplastic, at least once to demonstrate resolution or stability. If you choose this option, it is recommended that a reasonable interval is chosen. This might be 6 months for an asymptomatic woman.) This approach recognizes that sonographic follow-up may still be indicated if clinical circumstances necessitate.

As noted previously, some unilocular smooth-walled cysts cannot be categorized as being very likely to be non-neoplastic or very likely to be a benign neoplasm based on the sonographic evaluation thus far. The sonologist does not know with reasonable certainty what the mass is. The practical approach is then to ask if there a test or strategy that has a reasonable chance of enabling the sonologist to distinguish between these two possibilities and make a difference in the care of the patient. In such cases, sonographic follow-up will allow assessment of the stability or growth of the mass that may facilitate making the distinction. Obviously, if the mass resolves or is demonstrably smaller on follow-up, it is a non-neoplastic cyst which won't need treatment; conversely, if the mass grows, the suspicion that it is a benign neoplasm increases (though non-neoplastic cysts can also increase in size), likely to require intervention [Fig. 8].

If a unilocular smooth-walled cyst does not change in size on follow-up, it is more likely to be a non-neoplastic cyst, assuming that there has been enough of an interval between the two studies to enable detection of growth. Thus, it is important that follow-up studies be performed with enough of an interval to assist the sonologist in making this determination. It is common for sonologists encountering a unilocular smooth-walled cyst to recommend follow-up in 6 to 8 weeks or after one or two menstrual cycles. No doubt, the vast majority of non-neoplastic cysts in premenopausal women can be expected to change (get smaller or resolve) in that time-frame; in fact, most will resolve during the course of a single menstrual cycle (3 to 5 weeks).

Nevertheless, one should avoid the temptation to request sonographic follow-up at too short an interval for the follow-up to be meaningful. Universal application of the "6-to-8 weeks" rule for follow-up is inappropriate, especially in postmenopausal or perimenopausal women but also for many premenopausal women. Though non-neoplastic cysts in perimenopausal or postmenopausal woman are not uncommon and often self-limiting, there should be no expectation for these cysts to resolve or meaningfully change in 6 to 8 weeks. Furthermore, the asymptomatic premenopausal woman with a unilocular smooth-walled cyst is not well-served by the follow-up study performed in 6 to 8 weeks that again shows the cyst unchanged in size, as the time interval is too small to make any conclusions; it could still be a non-neoplastic cyst or a benign neoplasm. Granted, most cysts in premenopausal women will indeed resolve in this short interval, but documenting such resolution so quickly is usually not necessary, and the occasional non-neoplastic cyst will take more time to resolve.

In my practice, when I am trying to distinguish between a non-neoplastic cyst and a benign neoplasm as the cause of a typical unilocular smooth-walled anechoic ovarian cyst, I will request sonographic follow-up in 6 months. If there is some atypical feature that I suspect is artifactual or caused by a physiologic process (see ensuing discussion), or if there are even vague clinical symptoms possibly attributed to the mass, I will cut the follow-up interval in half (3 months). In the uncommon situation in which I am even more concerned about the atypical features of the mass but do not feel other testing or intervention is yet justified, or if there

are clinical symptoms clearly attributed to the mass which persist, I will further cut the follow-up interval in half (1.5 months, or 6 weeks).

When following a unilocular smooth-walled cyst to try to distinguish between a non-neoplastic cyst and a benign neoplasm, actual calculation of the volume of the cyst and the apparent doubling time can be helpful [see Fig. 8]. Small differences in the measured transverse, craniocaudal, and anteroposterior diameter of a cyst can occur between studies due to technical variability, so reliance on only one plane of measurement when serially imaging a mass can be misleading. Furthermore, small masses can demonstrate significant increase in volume with seemingly minimal diameter changes. For example, a cystic mass that is 2.0 cm in average diameter has doubled in size when the diameter increases to 2.5 cm. The formula for calculation of the volume of an ellipsoid mass (length × width × height × 0.52) is applied. To calculate the estimated doubling time, the time interval between the two measurements is divided by the percent increase in size of the mass. Thus, a cyst that grows from 3.5-cm average diameter to 4.0-cm average diameter in 6 months has an estimated doubling time of 1 year. This would be consistent with a benign neoplasm, and subsequent management would be appropriately directed with this assumption.

A unilocular cyst that demonstrates an increase in size is not always a benign neoplasm rather than a non-neoplastic cyst. Confidence in the assessment of interval growth depends on the magnitude of the change in measurement and the interval of observation. Re-evaluation of the size of a mass in a short interval allows technical variability to potentially mislead the observer. For example, a 2.0-cm average diameter mass that is subsequently reevaluated in 6 weeks and that appears to measure 2.1 cm in average diameter has potentially demonstrated a 15% increase in volume, resulting in a calculated doubling time of 40 weeks (6 weeks/0.15 = 40 weeks); obviously, this doubling time calculation is imprecise and unreliable because the magnitude of the measurement change (1 mm) is within the range of technical variability and the interval of observation is small. Even when the observer is more confident regarding the existence of true interval growth, an enlarging unilocular smooth-walled cyst could still be a non-neoplastic cyst rather than a benign neoplasm. Though there is no scientific literature to indicate the range of growth of benign ovarian cystic neoplasms, if the calculated doubling time of a unilocular smooth-walled cyst is very lengthy (exceeding 3 years), the mass could well be non-neoplastic. Nevertheless, unless the calculated doubling time is very lengthy, it is reasonable to conclude that the enlarging unilocular

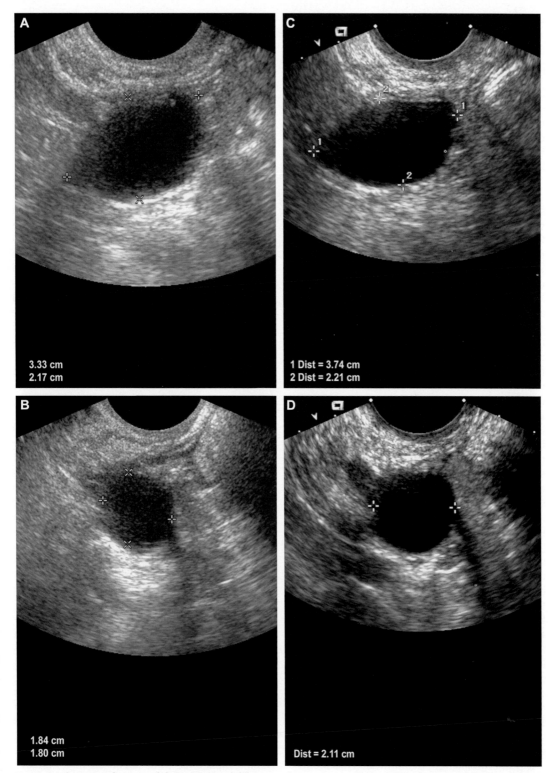

Fig. 8. Benign cystadenoma. (*A*) Sagittal and (*B*) coronal sonograms of the right ovary in a postmenopausal woman demonstrate a unilocular smooth-walled cyst measuring 3.3 × 2.2 × 1.8 cm. With these measurements, the volume of the cyst is calculated at 6.8 cubic cm. Subsequent follow-up sagittal (*C*) and coronal (*D*) sonograms performed 6 months later demonstrate the cyst to measure 3.7 × 2.2 × 2.1 cm. This yields a volume calculation of 8.9 cubic cm. The doubling time is calculated to be 19 months. A benign neoplasm was suspected; the mass was surgically removed and proved to be a serous cystadenoma.

smooth-walled cyst is a benign neoplasm and not a non-neoplastic cyst and manage the mass with this expectation. Once the cyst has demonstrated growth, the institution of other testing (including serologic CA-125 assessment or MRI) will not be clinically meaningful as the results will not allow one to conclude that the cyst is an atypical non-neoplastic cyst. Furthermore, it makes no clinical difference whether the enlarging cyst is a benign neoplasm or a non-neoplastic cyst; in either case, intervention is usually warranted.

Physiologic causes of findings that may raise concern

What if a mass violates one or more of the criteria for designation as a unilocular smooth-walled anechoic cyst? For example, suppose the mass contains a possible or definite septation, has wall irregularity or nodularity, or has diffuse or focal areas of echogenicity? For such lesions, the next step in the practical approach is to determine if the aberrant observation(s) could potentially be caused by a physiologic process. There are three physiologic processes to consider: (1) occurrence of two or more individual cysts next to each other, thus mimicking a multilocular mass with intervening septations; (2) cyst involution resulting in wall irregularity; and (3) intracystic hemorrhage resulting in internal echoes, internal strands and retractile clot. Of these three processes, hemorrhage is the most common in premenopausal women.

Hemorrhagic ovarian cysts frequently demonstrate features that can be confused with ovarian neoplasms [9]. Retracting thrombus adhering to the cyst wall may be mistaken for a mural nodule [Fig. 9]. Hemorrhagic cysts contain fine networks of linear echoes, which may be mistaken for "septations" [see Fig. 4]. True septations, when seen, are highly characteristic of ovarian neoplasms. Thus, this appearance may confuse the examiner into believing that the sonographically observed mass is a neoplasm. These fine linear echoes are not septations but rather a manifestation of clot architecture, likely originating from strands or bands of fibrin. It is probably because of these potentially confusing appearances that some older studies on hemorrhagic cysts most often conclude that they have a "nonspecific appearance," considering the diagnosis "difficult" and describing these masses as "the great imitator" [20].

It is unfortunate that hemorrhagic cysts are frequently said to be indistinguishable from ovarian neoplasms. In fact, hemorrhagic cysts almost always represent non-neoplastic cysts that will resolve spontaneously [21,22]. All of the 24 cases followed by Okai and colleagues [22] resolved within 8 weeks. Thirty percent of the masses resolved within 2 weeks. Among 38 surgically excised hemorrhagic cysts, none were neoplasms [21]. Importantly, no ovarian malignancies have been erroneously reported to represent hemorrhagic ovarian cysts in series evaluating the diagnostic performance of sonography for this pathologic entity. Therefore, if the examiner can correctly conclude that an ovarian mass is a hemorrhagic cyst, then one may be confident that the lesion will almost certainly resolve spontaneously. Should the lesion not resolve, there is virtually no chance that it represents a misdiagnosed ovarian carcinoma.

In contrast to the "nonspecific appearance" often previously described in the literature, our study indicates that hemorrhagic ovarian cysts have a very specific appearance in the vast majority (90%) of cases [9]. The key gray-scale ultrasound features to observe are the presence of fibrin strands or retracting clot, with absence of suspected septations and wall irregularity secondary helpful findings [see Fig. 4; Fig. 9]. When a unilocular smooth-walled cyst containing fibrin strands is identified, the observed mass is 200 times more likely to be a hemorrhagic ovarian cyst than any other possibility. Even if the sonologist can only be confident that fibrin strands are present but is uncertain as to whether there are coexisting true septations or wall irregularity, the presence of fibrin strands makes the mass 40 times more likely to be a hemorrhagic ovarian cyst [Fig. 10]. Finally, if one can identify a mural-based structure with features characteristic of a retracting clot, the mass is at least 67 times more likely to be a hemorrhagic ovarian cyst than any other entity. Understanding that the likelihood ratio is this high with these observations should help the less experienced sonologist feel more confident in the diagnosis and allow for observation instead of surgical intervention in appropriate cases. It is critical, therefore, for the sonologist to master the typical appearance of fibrin strands and retracting clot.

Jain and colleagues [23] described the appearance of fibrin strands in hemorrhagic cysts as "fish netting." Although a mass may contain many septations, the number is usually fewer than 20. In contrast, fibrin strands are often innumerable. Septations are usually thicker and more reflective than fibrin strands. Importantly, septations visually track for a reasonable and appropriate distance as they are viewed using real-time sonography. Indeed, even on still images, this feature is usually obvious. Unlike septations, fibrin strands are discontinuous and seem to flit from plane to plane either on real-time examination or on captured still images.

Similarly, retracting thrombus has a detectably and reliably different appearance than mural nodules. Mural nodules have convex margins, whereas

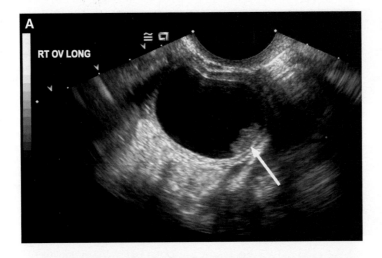

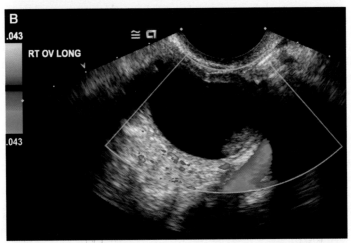

Fig. 9. Hemorrhagic ovarian cyst. (*A*) Sonogram of the right ovary in a premenopausal woman shows clumped material along the wall of an otherwise smooth-walled unilocular cyst at the 5 o'clock position. This retracting clot (*arrow*) has a slightly lower echogenicity than the adjacent wall. (*B*) Color Doppler sonogram of the cyst shows no detectable blood flow within the clot.

retracting thrombus has concave margins. Neoplastic tissue does not grow with a concave margin. Furthermore, echoes returning from thrombus tend to differ in amplitude compared with the cyst wall and are usually less echogenic. Mural nodules tend to have the same echogenicity as the cyst wall or, in the case of the Rochitansky nodule of cystic teratomas, markedly greater echogenicity than the cyst wall.

Color Doppler analysis is important to apply when one is considering the possibility of hemorrhage as a cause for apparent intracyst septations or cyst wall irregularity or nodularity. Retracting clot causing apparent septations or wall nodules should not exhibit blood flow [see Figs. 9 and 10]. Similarly, identification of vascularity within a mass

with diffuse low-level echoes identifies the mass as solid, not possibly cystic with internal hemorrhage. If one is entertaining the notion of hemorrhage as a cause for an aberrant finding, the demonstration of blood flow in that structure eliminates that possibility.

Unfortunately, the same cannot be said for the other physiologic processes that might possibly account for observations of apparent septations or wall irregularity. When two cysts lie next to each other, the resulting interface of cyst wall and any intervening ovarian parenchyma can be interpreted as a septation [Fig. 11]. Blood flow may be demonstrated within this "septation" as a function of the normal ovarian parenchyma "trapped" between the two cysts. Likewise, when physiologic cysts

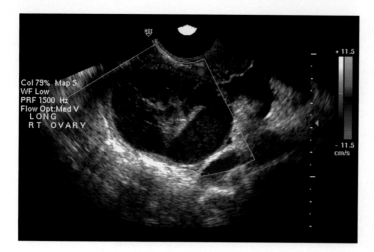

Fig. 10. Hemorrhagic ovarian cyst. Sonogram of the right ovary in a premenopausal woman, with color Doppler, shows a mass with internal echoes and linear echogenic bands which simulate septations. Fibrin strands are identified in one quadrant of the mass (from 6 to 9 o'clock). Color Doppler evaluation confirms the absence of demonstrable blood flow within the mass. The mass resolved on follow-up sonogram performed 6 weeks later.

involute, the wall irregularity of the cyst, corresponding to normal ovarian parenchyma along the surface of the flaccid cyst, can contain vessels.

Once the sonologist has determined that a physiologic process (adjacent cyst, cyst involution, or intracyst hemorrhage) could possibly account for the observations that make the mass not be classified as a unilocular anechoic smooth-walled cyst, he or she makes a general assessment of how likely it is that the mass will prove to be non-neoplastic in the same manner as described previously for the unilocular smooth-walled anechoic cyst. Again, factors to consider will include growth rate, location, patient hormonal status, and cyst size. Because of the compelling likelihood that one is dealing with a non-neoplastic hemorrhagic cyst with some observations (fibrin strands and retracting clot), it is reasonable to ignore those hemorrhagic cysts that contain these characteristic features when they are below the 4 cm size threshold articulated previously (assuming that the patient becomes asymptomatic); in such cases, sonographic reports should emphasize that sonographic follow-up may not be necessary. In other cases, sonographic follow-up allows assessment of cyst resolution, stability, or growth, to help distinguish between a non-neoplastic cyst and other possible causes of the mass. In this situation, the time interval chosen for follow-up is often justifiably shorter than the 6-month period chosen for the asymptomatic unilocular smooth-walled anechoic cyst. As articulated previously, I usually choose to cut the follow-up interval in half (3 months instead of 6 months) when there is a finding potentially caused by a physiologic process or even by another half (i.e., 1.5 months, or 6 weeks) when I think a particularly ominous sonographic finding might possibly be caused by hemorrhage or cyst involution.

One final comment regarding hemorrhage and cyst involution as a cause of wall irregularity; these physiologic processes occur almost exclusively in premenopausal women. It would be extremely unusual for intracyst hemorrhage to result in retractile clot in a woman who has undergone menopause, and these women would not be expected to have an involuting corpus luteum cyst. Of course, the coexistence of two unilocular cysts next to each other, simulating a single multilocular cyst, can occur in women of any age.

When physiologic process is unlikely, has a characteristic pattern been established?

The mass that is not a unilocular anechoic smooth-walled cyst, due to features that are not possibly physiologic in origin, is then analyzed to determine if features characteristic of a particular category have been observed. The categories for a cystic mass to consider would include non-neoplastic cyst, endometrioma, hydrosalpinx, peritoneal inclusion cyst, benign cystic neoplasm, cystic teratoma, and cystic malignancy. For each of these categories, specific observations can enable the sonologist to reasonably conclude that the mass in question is caused by that entity.

Non-neoplastic cyst

Most non-neoplastic cysts will have already been identified as such by the preceding analysis of unilocularity, wall regularity, and likely physiologic mimics of suspicious pathology. Nevertheless, some cysts will not meet these preceding criteria but can still be confidently assumed to be non-neoplastic by demonstrating lack of interval growth [Fig. 12]. Thus, the cyst which appears to have wall irregularity not due to hemorrhage (because the

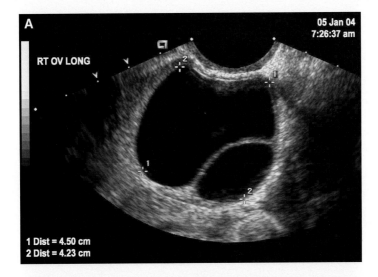

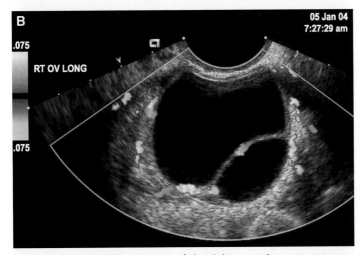

Fig. 11. Two adjacent unilocular cysts. (*A*) Sonogram of the right ovary in a premenopausal woman shows an apparent septation between two cystic compartments. Although this could be a bilocular cyst with an internal septation, the sonologist needs to consider that it could reasonably also be two adjacent unilocular cysts (as it was in this case). (*B*) Color Doppler sonogram demonstrates blood flow in the possible septation between the two cystic compartments. Normal ovarian parenchyma trapped between two unilocular cysts (as in this case) can demonstrate blood flow.

irregularity has not resolved) could still be classified as likely due to a non-neoplastic cyst by demonstrating no growth with serial sonography over a sufficiently long observation interval (at least 2 years). Having established this stability, the mass can then be managed in a manner appropriate for a non-neoplastic cyst. This would include continued periodic sonographic re-evaluation, percutaneous aspiration with or without sclerotherapy or methotrexate injection, or surgical removal.

Endometrioma

The presence of diffuse low-level internal echoes is an important feature that helps to consider the possibility of endometrioma as the cause of an

adnexal mass; our prior study demonstrated that 95% of endometriomas exhibit diffuse low-level internal echoes, with technical factors likely accounting for those few endometriomas in which low-level echoes were not demonstrated [Fig. 13] [8]. While the absence of this finding does not exclude endometrioma, it significantly decreases the likelihood of that diagnosis (negative likelihood ratio = 0.1). Nevertheless, the presence of diffuse low-level echoes in a mass is clearly not enough for the sonologist to conclude that the mass is an endometrioma, as some hemorrhagic ovarian cysts, benign neoplasms (including cystic teratoma), and malignancies can also exhibit this feature [Fig. 14].

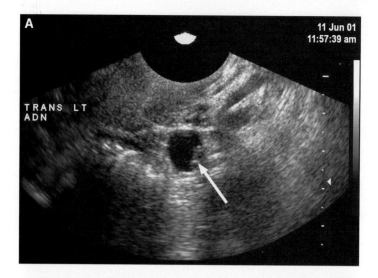

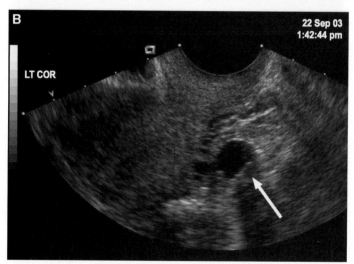

Fig. 12. Non-neoplastic cyst with wall irregularity. (*A*) Sonogram of the left ovary in a postmenopausal woman shows a small 1-cm cyst with wall irregularity (*arrow*). Color Doppler images (not shown) did not demonstrate blood flow in the area of focal wall irregularity. (*B*) The cyst was periodically followed with ultrasound. Follow-up sonogram 2 years later demonstrates no change in the size or appearance of the cyst or focal area of irregularity (*arrow*). The mass is likely a non-neoplastic cyst and is justifiably further managed conservatively.

As discussed previously, hemorrhagic cysts are almost exclusively non-neoplastic and most resolve spontaneously; they are surgically removed only when patients have compelling acute symptoms. The practical approach to the adnexal mass articulated thus far allows the sonographer to consider the possibility that a physiologic process (intracyst hemorrhage in a premenopausal woman) is the cause for the diffuse internal echoes in an otherwise unilocular smooth-walled mass. This justifiably leads to follow-up sonography as a diagnostic strategy to use to distinguish between acute hemorrhagic cyst and endometrioma [see Fig. 14]. If the diffuse low-level echoes persist unchanged on the follow-up examination, acute hemorrhagic cyst can be reasonably excluded from consideration.

Another particularly helpful observation to enable distinction between the acute hemorrhagic cyst and the endometrioma is the presence of one or more hyperechoic foci in the wall of a unilocular smooth-walled cyst with diffuse low-level echoes [see Fig. 13]. In our study, hyperechoic wall foci were seen in only 1 of 69 non-neoplastic cysts (a mass that did not resolve with periodic sonographic follow-up and considered a "simple" cyst at pathology) but were found in 14 of 40 (35%) endometriomas [8]. Based on these data, a smooth-walled mass with low-level internal echoes and

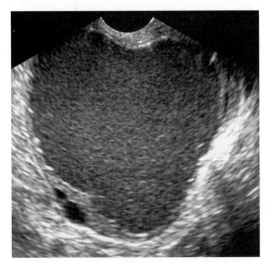

Fig. 13. Endometrioma. Sonogram of the left ovary shows a mass with diffuse low-level internal echoes and multiple hyperechoic wall foci (best seen at 8 to 9 o'clock).

coexisting hyperechoic wall foci is 32 times more likely to be an endometrioma than another adnexal mass; for masses that exhibit this pattern, sonographic follow-up is a low-yield course of action.

The pathologic basis of these hyperechoic wall foci has not been established. Given the similarity in appearance to hyperechoic wall foci seen in the gallbladder wall in patients with hyperplastic cholecystoses, due to the presence of cholesterol within polyps or Rokitansky-Aschoff sinuses, it has been postulated that these foci may contain cholesterol, perhaps from the breakdown of cell membranes subsequently phagocytized by giant cells. This may explain why they are seen in endometriomas, which contain chronic collections of cells that have had time to break down, and are not seen in

spontaneously resolving lesions such as acute hemorrhagic cysts.

The presence of hyperechoic wall foci in a cystic mass allows the observer to discount the possibility that the mass will resolve with expectant management. It does not necessarily mean that the mass is an endometrioma, however; if the theory that these hyperechoic wall foci represent cholesterol deposition in the wall of a "chronic" mass is true, one could also expect to see these hyperechoic foci in neoplasms. Indeed, neoplasms can exhibit this feature [8].

Thus, to have confidence that a mass with diffuse low-level echoes is an endometrioma, there is considerable benefit from further assessment of wall nodularity, a feature that is associated with neoplasia [24]. In our prior study, excluding masses with wall nodularity from the diagnosis of endometrioma helped to distinguish the endometriomas from neoplasms, especially malignancies [8]. However, as 20% of endometriomas can demonstrate wall nodularity, one can expect to be unable to reasonably distinguish between neoplasm and endometrioma for some masses with diffuse low-level echoes [Fig. 15]. Of the 11 masses in our study that demonstrated low-level internal echoes with wall nodularity but no features of cystic teratoma, 6 were endometriomas and 5 were neoplasms. This subgroup of patients may benefit from additional imaging with color Doppler sonography or MRI to try to distinguish between neoplastic and non-neoplastic causes of wall nodularity.

Hydrosalpinx

Sonographic findings associated with hydrosalpinx have been described by multiple investigators. Tessler and colleagues [25] found a tubular structure with folded configuration (incomplete septation)

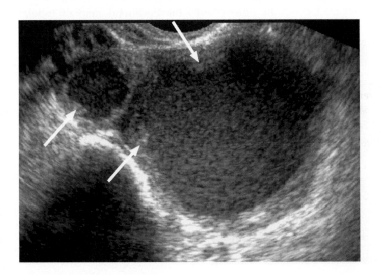

Fig. 14. Two hemorrhagic ovarian cysts. Sonogram of the right ovary in a premenopausal woman shows two masses with diffuse low level-internal echoes. Both cysts show mild wall irregularity (*arrows*). Both hemorrhagic cysts resolved on follow-up sonography performed 3 months later.

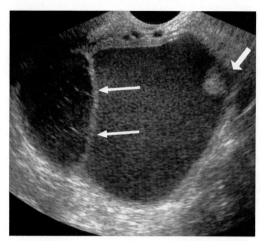

Fig. 15. Endometrioma with wall nodule. Sonogram of the left ovary shows a cystic compartment with diffuse low-level internal echoes and wall nodule (*thick arrow*). It is uncertain based on this image whether the entire mass is bilocular with an internal septation (*thin arrows*) or whether there are two adjacent cysts with intervening ovarian parenchyma. A small amount of normal ovarian parenchyma containing three follicles is present at the 12 o'clock position. At pathologic evaluation after laparoscopic surgical removal, no wall vegetations were identified; the apparent wall nodule was likely related to clot fibrosis.

as the most consistent feature in their 12 cases of hydrosalpinx [Fig. 16]. Short linear projections were also seen in approximately half of their patients. Timor-Tritsch and colleagues [26] expanded the analysis of the sonographic features of hydrosalpinx by analyzing the mass shape, wall structure, wall thickness, and extent of ovarian involvement. This analysis suggested that many hydrosalpinges were ovoid or pear-shaped fluid collections containing incomplete septa, short linear projections ("cogwheel" sign), or small hyperechoic mural nodules ("beads-on-a-string").

Recent data have refined these observations [11]. The most accurate sonographic diagnosis of hydrosalpinx as the cause of a cystic adnexal mass is achieved by first determining whether or not the mass appears tubular and then focusing on whether a waist sign or small round projections can be identified [see Fig. 16; Fig. 17]. The small round projections correspond to the "beads-on-a-string" described by Timor-Tritsch and colleagues [26], pathologically caused by fibrosis of endosalpingeal folds. The waist sign refers to diametrically opposed indentations along the wall of the mass.

As we recently reported [11], in our experience the combination of tubular shape and waist sign had no false positives for diagnosis of hydrosalpinx, leading to a calculated likelihood ratio exceeding 18.9; the exact likelihood ratio falls somewhere between this value and infinity (more precise determination of the true likelihood ratio of this combination of findings for the diagnosis of hydrosalpinx would have required a larger study population leading to at least one false-positive case). The combination of tubular shape with small round mural projections also performed very well, with likelihood ratio of 22.1; there was one false positive case using this combination, in which a paratubal cyst exhibited both features.

Two of the previously described sonographic findings associated with hydrosalpinx had no additional value in predicting that a mass was a hydrosalpinx when combined with the observation of tubular shape. Although the presence of an incomplete septation and short linear projections were findings predictive of hydrosalpinx, each was less predictive than tubular shape or the waist sign; moreover, in contrast to the waist sign and small round projections, neither incomplete septation nor small linear projection improved diagnostic performance when combined with tubular shape. In other words, the likelihood ratio of tubular

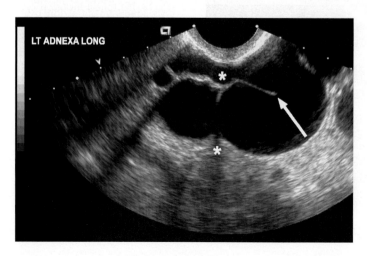

LT ADNEXA LONG

Fig. 16. Hydrosalpinx. Sonogram of the left adnexa shows a cystic mass with folded tubular configuration. The folded configuration leads to an apparent "incomplete septation" (*arrow*). There is a waist sign (*asterisks*), which refers to the presence of diametrically opposed indentations along the wall of the mass. A short linear projection is present at one of the sites of indentation.

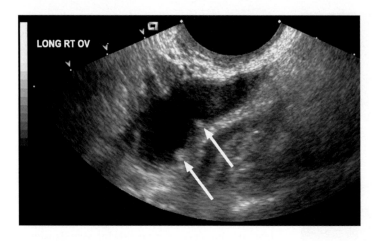

Fig. 17. Hydrosalpinx. Sonogram of the right adnexa shows a tubular cystic mass with small round projections along the wall (*arrows*), which have been described as "beads-on-a-string."

shape when combined with incomplete septation or short linear projection for the diagnosis of hydrosalpinx decreased as compared with the likelihood ratio of tubular shape alone. This is because apparent incomplete septations are also identified in some cystic neoplasms.

When trying to distinguish a hydrosalpinx from a cystic ovarian neoplasm, the sonographic identification of a normal-appearing ovary ipsilateral to a cystic adnexal mass has an extremely positive effect on the ability of the sonologist to accurately predict that the mass is a hydrosalpinx and not a cystadenoma or cystadenofibroma. Although paraovarian cystadenomas can occur, they are exceedingly rare. Thus, careful attention to identification of a normal ovary ipsilateral to the mass suspected of being a hydrosalpinx can clinch the diagnosis.

Peritoneal inclusion cyst

Peritoneal inclusion cysts, also known as peritoneal pseudocysts, occur as a result of trapped fluid between the ovary and adhesions in the peritoneal cavity. They begin in premenopausal patients who have had prior surgery, trauma, peritoneal infection, or endometriosis. The sonographic appearance of these peritoneal inclusion cysts can be pathognomonic [27]; in such cases, the margins of the cystic collection follow the contours of the pelvis, with some areas of acute angulation, and the often deformed ovary can be seen suspended among the adhesions centrally or peripherally [Fig. 18].

Cystic teratoma

A number of sonographic findings have been associated with cystic teratoma [10]. The feature that most commonly defines an ovarian mass as a cystic teratoma is the observation of focal or diffuse high-amplitude echoes that attenuate the acoustic beam (shadowing echodensity) [Fig. 19]. There are three types of tissues that can produce this finding: calcified structures like bone and teeth, clumps of hair in a cystic cavity, and fat in a Rokitansky protuberance. It does not matter which of the three situations

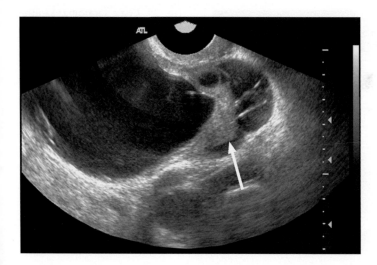

Fig. 18. Peritoneal inclusion cyst. Sonogram of the left adnexa shows a deformed ovary (*arrow*) with large exophytic cystic collection on one side, as well as smaller collection of fluid with thin septations on the other side.

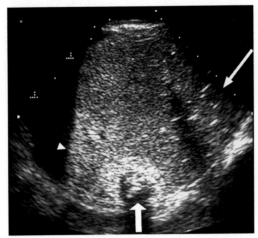

Fig. 19. Cystic teratoma. Sagittal endovaginal sonogram of an adnexal mass demonstrates shadowing echodensity (*thick arrow*), regional area of bright internal echoes (*arrowhead*), and hyperechoic lines and dots (*long arrow*). This combination of sonographic features is virtually pathognomonic for a cystic teratoma.

results in the sonographic identification of focal or diffuse high-amplitude echoes that attenuate the acoustic beam. Each of these tissues predicts that an ovarian mass is a cystic teratoma. Almost 90% of cystic teratomas demonstrate a shadowing echodensity; in only 16% of cases, there will be none of the other sonographic features associated with cystic teratomas [10].

There are two other important sonographic findings associated with dermoids [10]. The presence of diffuse or regional high-amplitude echoes within the mass, one of these other findings, is due to sebum; nearly 60% of cystic teratomas will exhibit this finding [see Fig. 19]. The other important

feature is the presence of hyperechoic lines and dots within the mass, the so-called "dermoid mesh" [28]. This sonographic appearance is caused by hair and is also found in about 60% of cystic teratomas [see Fig. 19].

Each of these three sonographic findings (shadowing echodensity, regional or diffuse bright echoes, hyperechoic lines and dots) can occasionally be identified or mimicked as isolated findings in other types of adnexal masses [10]. Fibrotic wall nodules seen in some endometriomas can produce acoustic shadowing. Hemorrhage can cause regional or diffuse mildly echogenic areas in a cystic mass. Fibrin strands in a hemorrhagic cyst can mimic the dermoid mesh. Amongst the three findings, the presence of a shadowing echodensity is the most accurate single feature enabling diagnosis of the mass as a cystic teratoma, with a likelihood ratio for dermoid exceeding 40 when only this feature is identified.

However, these findings become pathognomonic for identifying a cystic teratoma when they are seen in combination [10]. In our study [10] comparing cystic teratomas to nondermoid adnexal masses, 55 (76%) of the 72 dermoids exhibited two or more of these sonographic features, whereas none of the 178 nondermoids exhibited this feature set, resulting in a likelihood ratio exceeding 135. Thus, when sonologists identify any one of these sonographic findings, they can become highly confident regarding the diagnosis of cystic teratoma by carefully scrutinizing the mass for the presence of either of the other associated features [Fig. 20].

Benign and malignant cystic neoplasms (cystadenomas and cystadenocarcinomas)

The preceding discussion has analyzed some features of an adnexal mass that might enable the

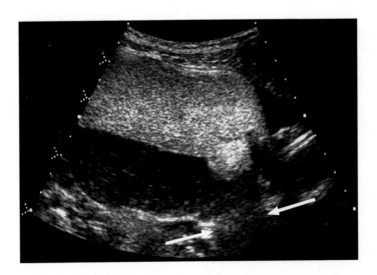

Fig. 20. Cystic teratoma. Sagittal transabdominal sonogram of an adnexal mass shows a large regional area of high-amplitude echoes. Additional scrutiny reveals a shadowing echodensity (*arrows* mark borders of the acoustic shadow). The presence of two features of cystic teratomas virtually assures that the mass is a dermoid.

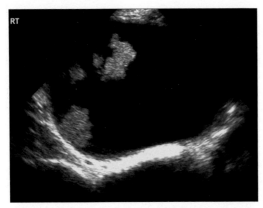

Fig. 21. Cystadenocarcinoma. Sonogram of the right adnexa reveals a cystic mass with large wall vegetations. Color Doppler evaluation showed obvious blood flow within the nodules (not shown). Surgical treatment and staging was performed by a gynecologic oncologist without additional imaging work-up.

sonologist to characterize the mass as a benign neoplasm, namely the unilocular smooth-walled cyst that is enlarging on follow-up examination. For these masses, the demonstration of interval growth is the key feature that enables the sonologist to confidently assert that the mass is not a typical non-neoplastic cyst, which would be expected to exhibit stability or resolution over time [see Fig. 8]. As noted previously, theoretically there may be an atypical non-neoplastic cyst that shows growth over time, at a rate that is indistinguishable from a benign neoplasm; nevertheless, trying to distinguish between a growing non-neoplastic cyst and a growing benign ovarian cystic neoplasm is usually not clinically relevant. Both masses merit surgical removal, and it is reasonable and practical to assume that the mass is a benign cystic neoplasm.

In this situation, further testing with serologic evaluation or MRI is unlikely to provide compelling additional data to distinguish between the rare enlarging non-neoplastic cyst and the benign neoplasm.

The presence of septations or mural or septal nodules in a cystic mass is compelling evidence that the mass is an ovarian neoplasm (benign or malignant) [Figs. 21 and 22] [29]. Benignancy is favored over malignancy when septations are smooth and relatively thin, and when the mural or septal nodularity is minor. Thick septations, irregular solid areas, poorly defined margins, and coexisting ascites or matted bowel loops are features highly specific but not very sensitive for malignancy [30]. As described previously, after considering and excluding the possibility that the aberrant findings could be reasonably caused by a physiologic process, the sonologist confronted with a mass exhibiting septations or mural nodularity can confidently indicate that the mass is a neoplasm. He or she may not be sure if the mass is benign or malignant in such cases; benignancy or malignancy may be favored based on the specific features of the case, but the sonologist may be confident of this assessment in only the most straightforward cases.

In keeping with the basic approach, the question to consider after identifying a neoplasm is whether any additional testing should be performed, recommended, or offered. The answer depends on whether it makes any difference. Serologic evaluation of CA-125 levels may help to implicate malignancy over benignancy. MRI may help to better demonstrate malignant-appearing features. These additional tests might be useful if the results would lead to a different surgical approach (or different surgeon) when the patient goes to surgery. Doppler analysis of the resistive index of flow in the wall of

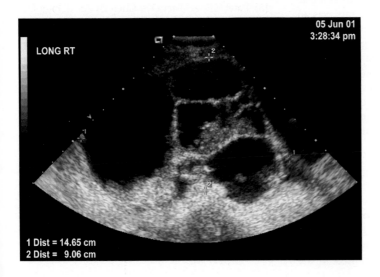

1 Dist = 14.65 cm
2 Dist = 9.06 cm

Fig. 22. Cystadenocarcinoma. Transabdominal sonogram of the right adnexa shows a large cystic and solid mass (demarcated with electronic calipers), with multiple septations, some harboring large septal nodules. The sonologist can confidently diagnose malignancy based on these features.

the mass has not been shown to have any reproducible accuracy in distinguishing benign from malignant cystic ovarian neoplasms [31] and cannot be recommended as a high-utility maneuver.

Other potentially characteristic adnexal masses

Other categories of adnexal pathology that have not yet been discussed are beyond the scope of this article. In some cases, there are characteristic features (both clinical and imaging) that enable confident classification of an adnexal masses into one of these categories, which include ectopic pregnancy, abscess/inflammatory mass, torsed ovary, exophytic leiomyoma, ovarian fibroma, and other solid mass.

Further imaging or surgical exploration

Using the algorithm as a practical approach to the adnexal mass, the sonologist should be able to confidently classify many, if not most, adnexal masses into one of the categories of suspected pathology: (1) non-neoplastic cyst; (2) hemorrhagic ovarian cyst; (3) endometrioma; (4) hydrosalpinx; (5) peritoneal inclusion cyst; (6) benign cystic neoplasm; (7) cystic teratoma; (8) cystic malignancy; (9) ectopic pregnancy; (10) abscess/inflammatory mass; (11) torsed ovary; (12) exophytic or broad ligament myoma; (13) ovarian fibroma; (14) solid mass. When the sonographic findings do not allow confidence in establishing one category, further testing with MRI can lead to additional observations that enable categorization. The endometrioma with apparently avascular wall nodularity, the atypical hydrosalpinx without sonographically identified adjacent ovary, and the peritoneal inclusion cyst in which the suspended ovary is not visible are some examples of masses that might benefit from further evaluation with MRI, since one might choose to not surgically evaluate the patient if one could be reasonably assured that the mass was an endometrioma, hydrosalpinx, or peritioneal pseudocyst. Similarly, establishing the diagnosis of exophytic leiomyoma or ovarian fibroma using MRI in those cases without characteristic sonographic observations would be useful to avoid surgical evaluation. Ultimately, if imaging is unable to characterize a mass into one of these categories using the suggested algorithm, diagnostic surgical exploration will be necessary.

Summary

Gynecologic sonography has matured into a highly effective and accurate tool enabling confident diagnosis of a variety of adnexal masses. Using a practical evidence-based approach, sonologists are well equipped to differentiate expected findings in the normal ovary from pathologic entities and can often generate specific conclusions regarding the cause of an adnexal mass. Mastery of the diagnostic strategies to use when an adnexal mass is identified and the sonographic patterns of various types of adnexal pathology contributes greatly to the proper and cost-effective care of a woman with an adnexal mass.

References

[1] Bakos O, Lundkvist O, Wide L, Bergh T. Ultrasonographical and hormonal description of the normal ovulatory menstrual cycle. Acta Obstet Gynecol Scand 1994;73:790–6.

[2] Ron-El R, Nachum H, Golan A, et al. Binovular human ovarian follicles associated with in vitro fertilization: incidence and outcome. Fertil Steril 1990;54:869–72.

[3] Pache TD, Wladimiroff JW, de Jong FH, et al. Growth patterns of nondominant ovarian follicles during the normal menstrual cycle. Fertil Steril 1990;54:638–42.

[4] Swire MN, Castro-Aragon I, Levine D. Various sonographic appearances of the hemorrhagic corpus luteum cyst. Ultrasound Q 2004;20:45–58.

[5] Timor-Tritsch IE, Goldstein SR. The complexity of a "complex mass" and the simplicity of a "simple cyst". J Ultrasound Med 2005;24:255–8.

[6] Timmerman D, Schwarzler P, Collins WP, et al. Subjective assessment of adnexal masses with the use of ultrasonography: an analysis of interobserver variability and experience. Ultrasound Obstet Gynecol 1999;13:11–6.

[7] Valentin L, Hagen B, Tingulstad S, Eik-Nes S. Comparison of "pattern recognition" and logistic regression models for discrimination between benign and malignant pelvic masses: a prospective cross validation. Ultrasound Obstet Gynecol 2001;18:357–65.

[8] Patel MD, Feldstein VA, Chen DC, et al. Endometriomas: diagnostic performance of US. Radiology 1999;210:739–45.

[9] Patel MD, Feldstein VA, Filly RA. The likelihood ratio of sonographic findings for the diagnosis of hemorrhagic ovarian cysts. J Ultrasound Med 2005;24:607–15.

[10] Patel MD, Feldstein VA, Lipson SD, et al. Cystic teratomas of the ovary: diagnostic value of sonography. AJR Am J Roentgenol 1998;171:1061–5.

[11] Patel MD, Acord DL, Young SW. Likelihood ratio of sonographic findings in discriminating hydrosalpinx from other adnexal masses. AJR 2006; 186.

[12] Nardo LG, Kroon ND, Reginald PW. Persistent unilocular ovarian cysts in a general population of postmenopausal women: is there a place for expectant management? Obstet Gynecol 2003; 102:589–93.

[13] Modesitt SC, Pavlik EJ, Ueland FR, et al. Risk of malignancy in unilocular ovarian cystic tumors less than 10 centimeters in diameter. Obstet Gynecol 2003;102:594–9.

[14] Dorum A, Blom GP, Ekerhovd E, Granberg S. Prevalence and histologic diagnosis of adnexal cysts in postmenopausal women: an autopsy study. Am J Obstet Gynecol 2005;192:48–54.

[15] Ekerhovd E, Wienerroith H, Staudach A, Granberg S. Preoperative assessment of unilocular adnexal cysts by transvaginal ultrasonography: a comparison between ultrasonographic morphologic imaging and histopathologic diagnosis. Am J Obstet Gynecol 2001;184:48–54.

[16] Mesogitis S, Daskalakis G, Pilalis A, et al. Management of ovarian cysts with aspiration and methotrexate injection. Radiology 2005;235:668–73.

[17] Timmerman D, Bourne TH, Tailor A, et al. A comparison of methods for preoperative discrimination between malignant and benign adnexal masses: the development of a new logistic regression model. Am J Obstet Gynecol 1999;181:57–65.

[18] Korbin CD, Brown DL, Welch WR. Paraovarian cystadenomas and cystadenofibromas: sonographic characteristics in 14 cases. Radiology 1998;208:459–62.

[19] Ghossain MA, Braidy CG, Kanso HN, et al. Extra-ovarian cystadenomas: ultrasound and MR findings in 7 cases. J Comput Assist Tomogr 2005;29: 74–9.

[20] Bass IS, Haller JO, Friedman AP, et al. The sonographic appearance of the hemorrhagic ovarian cyst in adolescents. J Ultrasound Med 1984;3: 509–13.

[21] Baltarowich OH, Kurtz AB, Pasto ME, et al. The spectrum of sonographic findings in hemorrhagic ovarian cysts. AJR Am J Roentgenol 1987; 148:901–5.

[22] Okai T, Kobayashi K, Ryo E, et al. Transvaginal sonographic appearance of hemorrhagic functional ovarian cysts and their spontaneous regression. Int J Gynaecol Obstet 1994;44:47–52.

[23] Jain KA, Friedman DL, Pettinger TW, et al. Adnexal masses: comparison of specificity of endovaginal US and pelvic MR imaging. Radiology 1993;186:697–704.

[24] Sassone AM, Timor-Tritsch IE, Artner A, et al. Transvaginal sonographic characterization of ovarian disease: evaluation of a new scoring system to predict ovarian malignancy. Obstet Gynecol 1991;78:70–6.

[25] Tessler FN, Perrella RR, Fleischer AC, Grant EG. Endovaginal sonographic diagnosis of dilated fallopian tubes. AJR 1989;153:523–5.

[26] Timor-Tritsch IE, Lerner JP, Monteagudo A, Murphy KE, Heller DS. Transvaginal sonographic markers of tubal inflammatory disease. Ultrasound Obstet Gynecol 1998;12:56–66.

[27] Jain KA. Imaging of peritoneal inclusion cysts. AJR Am J Roentgenol 2000;174:1559–63.

[28] Malde HM, Kedar RP, Chadha D, Nayak S. Dermoid mesh: a sonographic sign of ovarian teratoma. AJR Am J Roentgenol 1992;159: 1349–50.

[29] Granberg S, Wikland M, Jansson I. Macroscopic characterization of ovarian tumors and the relation to the histological diagnosis: criteria to be used for ultrasound evaluation. Gynecol Oncol 1989;35:139–44.

[30] Herrmann UJ Jr, Locher GW, Goldhirsch A. Sonographic patterns of ovarian tumors: prediction of malignancy. Obstet Gynecol 1987;69: 777–81.

[31] Levine D, Feldstein VA, Babcook CJ, Filly RA. Sonography of ovarian masses: poor sensitivity of resistive index for identifying malignant lesions. AJR Am J Roentgenol 1994;162:1355–9.

ELSEVIER SAUNDERS

RADIOLOGIC
CLINICS
OF NORTH AMERICA

Radiol Clin N Am 44 (2006) 901–910

Abnormal Uterine Bleeding: The Role of Ultrasound

Steven R. Goldstein, MD

- Evolution of endometrial assessment
- Transvaginal ultrasound
- Other considerations for sonohysterography
  Timing of the procedure
  Difficulty threading the catheter
- *Anesthesia/analgesia*
- *Risk of infection*
- Concern about spreading adenocarcinoma into the peritoneal cavity
- Inadequate distension of the cavity
- Summary
- References

Abnormal uterine bleeding accounts for up to 20% of gynecologic visits [1]. Any pregnancy event must first be excluded, and the use of inexpensive, rapid, monoclonal antibody urine human chorionic gonadotropin tests, readily available over-the-counter, makes this a relatively simple maneuver. When a pregnancy event has been excluded, the most likely cause of bleeding is dysfunctional anovulatory bleeding—what patients are often told is a "hormone imbalance." As women get older, however, organic pathology such as polyp, submucous myomas, hyperplasias, and even frank carcinoma become more likely. According to the SEER database [2], the incidence of endometrial carcinoma in women aged 30 to 34 years is 2.3/100,000, increases to 6.1/100,000 between ages 35 and 40 years, and rises dramatically to 36.2/100,000 in women aged 40 to 49 years. In postmenopausal women on no hormone replacement therapy, any bleeding is considered "cancer until proven otherwise," although the incidence of malignancy in such patients ranges from 2% to 10% depending on risk factors [3].

The role of the clinician in a patient who presents with bleeding is twofold: first, to exclude endometrial carcinoma in women older than 40 years [4],

and second, to identify the source of bleeding so it can be stopped or managed.

Most patients who have abnormal bleeding will have dysfunctional uterine bleeding in association with episodes of anovulation (premenopausal) or endometrial atrophy (postmenopausal) that can best be managed hormonally or expectantly with reassurance. The main goal is to distinguish such patients from those who have organic pathologic conditions in a safe, painless, convenient manner.

Evolution of endometrial assessment

Initially, curettage was the "gold standard." First described in 1843 [5], its performance in the hospital became the most common operation performed on women in the world. As early as the 1950s, a review of 6907 curettage procedures [6] found the technique missed endometrial lesions in 10% of cases. Of these, 80% were polyps.

In the 1970s, vacuum-suction curettage devices allowed sampling without anesthesia in an office setting. The most popular was the Vabra aspirator (Berkeley Medevices, Berkeley, California). This device was found to be 86% accurate in diagnosing cancer [7]. Subsequently, less expensive, smaller,

This article was originally published in *Ultrasound Clinics* 1:2, April 2006.
New York University School of Medicine, 530 First Avenue, Suite 10N, New York, NY 10016, USA
E-mail address: steven.goldstein@med.nyu.edu

doi:10.1016/j.rcl.2006.10.018

less painful plastic catheters with their own internal pistons to generate suction became popular. One of these, the Pipelle device (Unimar, Wilton, Connecticut), was found to have similar efficacy but better patient acceptance compared with the Vabra aspirator [8].

Rodriguez and colleagues [9] did a pathologic study of 25 hysterectomy specimens. The percentage of endometrial surface sampled by the Pipelle device was 4% versus 41% for the Vabra aspirator.

In one widely publicized study [10], the Pipelle had a 97.5% sensitivity to detect endometrial cancer in 40 patients undergoing hysterectomy. The shortcoming of that study was that the diagnosis of malignancy was known before the performance of the specimen collection.

In another important study, Guido and colleagues [11] also studied the Pipelle biopsy in patients who had known carcinoma undergoing hysterectomy. Among 65 patients, a Pipelle biopsy provided tissue adequate for analysis in 63 (97%), but malignancy was detected in only 54 patients (83%). Of the 11 with false-negative results, 5 (8%) had disease confined to endometrial polyps and 3 (5%) had tumor localized to less than 5% of the surface area of the cavity. The surface area of the endometrial involvement in that study was 5% or less of the cavity in 3 of 65 (5%); 5% to 25% of the cavity in 12 of 65 (18%), of which the Pipelle missed four cases; 26% to 50% of the cavity in 20 of 65 (31%), of which the Pipelle missed four; and greater than 50% of the cavity in 30 of 65 patients (46%), of which the Pipelle missed none. These results provide great insight about the way endometrial carcinoma can be distributed over the endometrial surface or confined to a polyp. Because tumors localized in a polyp or a small area of endometrium may go undetected, the investigators in that study concluded that the "Pipelle is excellent for detecting global processes in the endometrium."

From these data, it seems that undirected sampling, whether through curettage or various types of suction aspiration, is often fraught with error, especially in cases in which the abnormality is not global but focal (polyps, focal hyperplasia, or carcinoma involving small areas of the uterine cavity).

Transvaginal ultrasound

Introduced in the mid-1980s, the vaginal probe uses higher frequency transducers in close proximity to the structure being studied. It yields a degree of image magnification that has been dubbed sonomicroscopy [12]. In the early 1990s, it was used in women who had postmenopausal bleeding to see if it could predict which patients lacked significant tissue and could avoid dilation and curettage or endometrial biopsy and its discomfort, expense, and risk [13,14]. Consistently, the finding of a thin, distinct endometrial echo 4 to 5 mm or less has been shown to effectively exclude significant tissue in women who have bleeding. It is unfortunate that the corollary is not nearly as helpful. The positive predictive value of an endometrial echo greater than 5 mm is not so useful, although in the author's experience, many clinicians have inappropriately used a thick echo on ultrasound as an indicator of pathology. Such inappropriate application of transvaginal ultrasound is especially worrisome in patients who have no bleeding and in whom the finding is incidental.

Endometrial thickness should be measured on a sagittal (long-axis) image of the uterus, and the measurement should be performed on the thickest portion of the endometrium, excluding the hypoechoic inner myometrium. It is a "double-thickness" measurement from basalis to basalis [15].

If fluid is present, then it is usually associated with cervical stenosis and atrophy [16]. The layers are measured separately and should be symmetric. It should be remembered that the endometrial cavity is a three-dimensional structure, and attempts must be made to image the entire cavity. Recognizing the potentially pivotal role of transvaginal ultrasound in diagnostic evaluation, a statement should be included in the report regarding the technical adequacy of the scan. A well-defined endometrial echo should be seen taking off from the endocervical canal [Fig. 1]. It should be distinct. Often, fibroids, previous surgery, marked obesity, or an axial uterus may make visualization suboptimal. If so, it is acceptable and appropriate to conclude "endometrial echo not well visualized" [Fig. 2]. In these cases, ultrasound cannot be relied on to exclude disease. The next step for such patients who have bleeding should be hysteroscopy or saline infusion sonohysterography depending on the skill set and preference of the physician and patient.

Although the use of fluid enhancement was described with abdominal ultrasound for uterine and tubal observations [17], it never gained widespread use. The introduction of the vaginal probe changed that practice considerably [18,19]. The use of fluid instillation into the uterus coupled with such high-resolution transvaginal probes allows tremendous diagnostic enhancement with an inexpensive, simple, well-tolerated office procedure (see the article by R.B. Goldstein elsewhere in this issue).

In a prospective pilot study, saline infusion sonohysterography was performed in 21 women who had abnormal perimenopausal uterine bleeding [20]. Of the 21 patients, 8 had obvious polypoid lesions [Fig. 3] and were triaged for operative

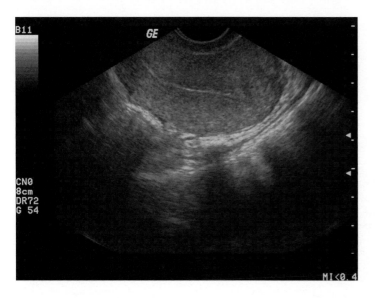

Fig. 1. Long-axis transvaginal ultrasound image of a postmenopausal patient who had a history of uterine bleeding. A thin, linear, distinct endometrial echo here has a negative predictive value of 99%. Notice that it is clearly seen taking off from the endocervical canal.

hysteroscopic removal. The pathology report confirmed benign polyps in all 8 patients. Three patients had submucous myomas. Two had wire-loop resectoscopic excision [Fig. 4]. The third, who had a submucous myoma that extended to the serosal edge of the uterus, received expectant management. Nine patients had no obvious anatomic lesion, and the endometrial thickness of the anterior or posterior wall was a maximum of 3.2 mm. The studies were purposely performed on days 4 to 6 of the bleeding cycle when early proliferative change would be expected if no anatomic abnormality existed. Biopsy in all 9 of these patients revealed early

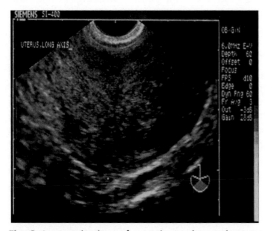

Fig. 2. Long-axis view of a patient who underwent previous uterine surgery in whom a meaningful distinct endometrial echo is technically inadequate. The clinician should never be afraid to state "endometrial echo not well visualized."

proliferative endometrium. Thus, these patients had dysfunctional (ie, anovulatory) uterine bleeding and were successfully treated with progestational agents. One patient had an endometrial thickness along the anterior wall of 7.6 mm, although the posterior wall was thin (2.3 mm). Curettage with hysteroscopy revealed simple hyperplasia without atypia; this patient was also treated with progestational agents. Thus, it was concluded that endometrial fluid instillation (sonohysterogram) to enhance vaginal ultrasonography in perimenopausal women can reliably distinguish between patients who have minimal tissue (3 mm or less single-layer measurements) whose bleeding is anovulatory and best treated hormonally from patients who have significant tissue (3 mm or more single-layer thickness) in need of formal curettage and hysteroscopy. Furthermore, polyps can be distinguished from submucous myomas. This distinction allows appropriate triage for operative hysteroscopy in terms of skill required and length of time and equipment needed. Furthermore, this procedure eliminates the need for diagnostic hysteroscopy in patients whose bleeding is dysfunctional.

As determined in this pilot study, the addition of saline infusion sonohysterography can reliably distinguish perimenopausal patients who have dysfunctional abnormal bleeding (no anatomic abnormality) from those who have globally thickened endometria or focal abnormalities.

A clinical algorithm was proposed and studied in a large prospective trial of perimenopausal women who had abnormal bleeding using unenhanced transvaginal ultrasonography followed by saline infusion sonohysterography for selected patients and

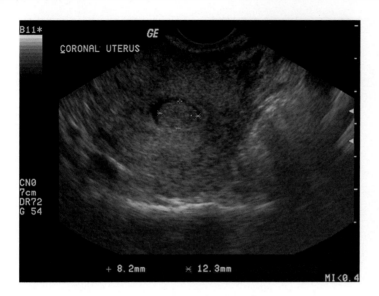

Fig. 3. Saline infusion sonohysterogram of a patient who had abnormal uterine bleeding. In this coronal view of the uterus, a polyp measuring 8.2 × 12.3 mm (*calipers*) is seen emanating from the posterior wall.

then no endometrial sampling, undirected endometrial sampling, or visually directed endometrial sampling depending on whether the ultrasonographically based triage revealed no anatomic abnormality, globally thickened endometrium, or focal abnormalities, respectively [Fig. 5] [21]. In that study, 280 patients (65%) displayed a thin, distinct, symmetric endometrial echo of 5 mm or less on days 4 to 6, and dysfunctional uterine bleeding was diagnosed. One hundred fifty-three (35%) had saline infusion sonohysterography. Of these procedures, 44 (29%) were performed because of the inability to adequately characterize and measure the endometrium [Fig. 6] and 109 (71%) were done for an endometrial measurement of 5 mm or greater. Sixty-one of those patients then had anterior and posterior endometrial thickness that was symmetric and less than 3 mm, compatible with dysfunctional uterine bleeding. Fifty-eight patients (13%) had focal polypoid masses [Fig. 7] that were removed hysteroscopically and confirmed pathologically. Twenty-two patients (5%) had submucous myomas, although 148 (34%) had clinical and ultrasonographic evidence of fibroids. Ten patients had symmetric single-layer measurements of endometrium at saline infusion sonohysterography greater than 3 mm (range, 3–9 mm). Of these, histologic type was proliferative endometrium in 5 and hyperplastic endometrium in 5. Saline infusion sonohysterography was technically inadequate in 2 patients who then underwent hysteroscopy with curettage. Undirected office biopsy alone without imaging potentially would have missed the diagnosis of focal lesions such as polyps, submucous myomas, and focal hyperplasia in up to 80 patients (18%).

Based on these results, it seems apparent that any "blind" endometrial sampling should be preceded by saline infusion sonohysterography if the endometrial thickness is greater than 5 mm. A process must be shown to be symmetrically "pan uterine" or global to justify a blind procedure. When changes are focal (eg, polyps, some hyperplasias, some carcinomas), they can be appreciated as such with fluid-instillation sonohysterography, and then directed biopsies must be performed.

In the pilot study [20], although 9 of 21 patients had obvious sonographic and clinical evidence of fibroids, only 3 had a submucous component. Six of 21 had intramural-subserosal myomas coexisting with dysfunctional uterine bleeding. In the large prospective study [21], 148 of 433 women had myomas but only 22 had a submucous component.

Usually, polyps are clearly discernable, as are submucous myomas. Sometimes, however, a broad-based polyp is difficult to distinguish from a submucosal myoma. This distinction may be important for preoperative triage, in that a truly pedunculated submucous myoma behaves more like a polyp in terms of skill and equipment required for its removal in the operating room, whereas a broad-based polyp may behave more like a myoma and require resectoscopic capability.

A reliable assessment with ultrasonography requires that the endometrial echo be homogeneous, that it is surrounded by an intact hypoechoic junctional zone, and that the operator constantly remembers that the endometrial cavity is a three-dimensional structure. This fact may account for why Dijkhuizen and colleagues [22] had four cases that supposedly measured less than 10

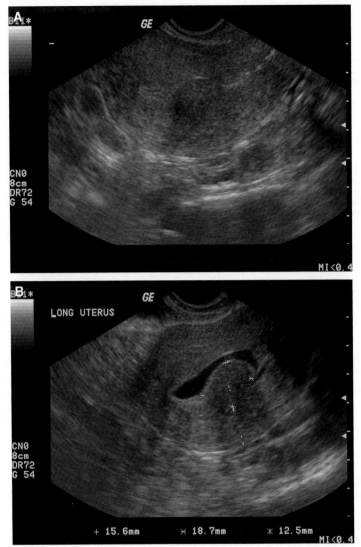

Fig. 4. (*A*) Long-axis view of a patient who had abnormal uterine bleeding. There is a central thickened uterine echo that is also heterogeneous. (*B*) Saline infusion sonohysterogram reveals an endoluminal mass (15.6 × 18.7 mm) outlined by calipers that represents an intraluminal myoma. Note the acoustic shadowing emanating from the myoma. Furthermore, note that the endometrial cavity itself is lined with thin endometrium compatible with the early proliferative phase in this perimenopausal patient. Finally, the distance from the back of the myoma to serosa is 12.5 mm (*calipers*).

mm (some as little as 2 mm) yet displayed polyps at hysteroscopy. Such cases underscore the importance of the three-dimensional character of the endometrial cavity and the occasional propensity of the ultrasonographic operator to obtain a limited number of two-dimensional views and assume that these represent the entire endometrial cavity. Any one "frozen" ultrasonographic image is nothing more than a two-dimensional "snapshot," and failure to meticulously recreate three-dimensional anatomy results in error.

New three-dimensional ultrasound equipment can eliminate errors that may occur when the operator does not pay meticulous attention to mentally recreating three-dimensional anatomy.

Furthermore, the use of color flow or power Doppler imaging to identify the central feeder vessel pathognomonic of an endometrial polyp is an alternative to sonohysterography in the diagnosis of polyps [Figs. 8 and 9]. This methodology had a positive predictive value of 81.3% in the study by Timmerman and colleagues [23].

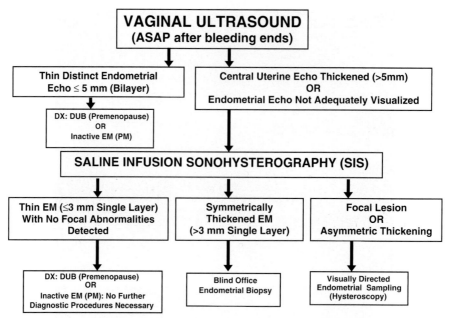

Fig. 5. Clinical algorithm for ultrasound-based triage of any patients who have abnormal uterine bleeding.

Other considerations for sonohysterography

Timing of the procedure

The uterus is an organ that has had multiple procedures in many women including D&C's, child birth, myomectomy, Caesarean sections, abortion, etc. As the endometrium proliferates it is not always a smooth homogeneous layer. Sonohysterography is best performed as soon as possible after the bleeding cycle has ended when the endometrium is as thin as it is going to be all month long. Otherwise focal irregularities in the contour of the endometrium may be mistaken for small polyps or focal areas of endometrial hyperplasia [Fig. 9]. This was supported in a prospective blinded study by Wolman and colleagues [24] in which there was a 27% false positive rate in sonohysterography performed from day 16 to 28, while there were none when the procedure was performed prior to day 10.

Sometimes the patient has such irregular bleeding that she can not tell what is an actual menses. It may be helpful in such cases to use an empiric course of a progestogen such as medroxyprogesterone acetate 10mg daily for 10 days as a "medical curettage" and then time the ultrasound evaluation to the withdrawal bleed.

Difficulty threading the catheter

Occasionally, there will be difficulty in threading the catheter into its desired position. Using the other hand to change the position of the speculum will often modify the angle of the cervix with the fundus sufficiently to allow successful completion. Use of a tenaculum is a last resort. A cervical stabilizer will be less painful, less traumatic and does not cause bleeding from the cervix.

Anesthesia/analgesia

Anesthesia or analgesia is not required. In more than 1000 cases, I have seen three cases of a vasovagal response reminiscent of those occasionally seen with a plastic intrauterine device insertion in a nulliparous patient. The sonohysterography catheter is 1.8 mm in diameter and is remarkably painless in its insertion. The procedure is extremely well tolerated with no pain in the overwhelming majority of patients and minimal cramping in a very few.

Risk of infection

Sonohysterography should be handled similarly to traditional HSG. Thus, the decision about whether to obtain gonorrhoea or Chlamydia cultures as well as whether to use antibiotics will depend very much on the patient population with which the physician normally deals. In my experience, I have not routinely obtained cultures for sexually transmitted diseases nor have prophylactic antibiotics been used. In more than 1000 cases, I have not experienced any infectious morbidity. Of 1,153 procedures performed [25] the incidence of infectious complications that require surgical resolution was 0.7% which is similar to diagnostic hysteroscopy [26] but less than hysterosalpingography [27].

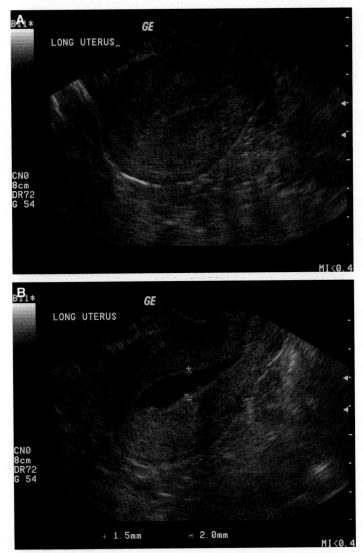

Fig. 6. (*A*) Transvaginal scan in long-axis view of a perimenopausal patient who had abnormal uterine bleeding. The endometrial echo is not sufficiently seen along its entirety to make an accurate diagnosis. (*B*) Saline infusion sonohysterography reveals a lack of any endoluminal mass. The anterior and posterior endometrium measure 1.5 and 2.0 mm, respectively (*calipers*).

Concern about spreading adenocarcinoma into the peritoneal cavity

Concern about spreading adenocarcinoma is a question of the benefit outweighing any theoretic risk [24–27]. It is no longer standard practice to tie the fallopian tubes with silk before a total abdominal hysterectomy and bilateral salpingo-oophorectomy for endometrial carcinoma. Furthermore, hysteroscopy with saline or other distending media would have the same theoretic concern. Survival rates of patients who had endometrial carcinoma and underwent standard HSG were not different between patients who demonstrated intraperitoneal spill of the contrast medium and patients who did not [28]. Alcazar and colleagues [29] performed sonohysterography on 14 consecutive patients who had stage I adenocarcinoma of the endometrium. It was done at the time of laparotomy just when the abdomen was opened but before the start of the surgical procedure. All 14 readily spilled saline from the fallopian tubes. The fluid was analyzed, as were the cell washings. Only 1 patient (7%) had malignant cells in the spilled fluid, causing the investigators to conclude that the risk of malignant cell dissemination exists but is small.

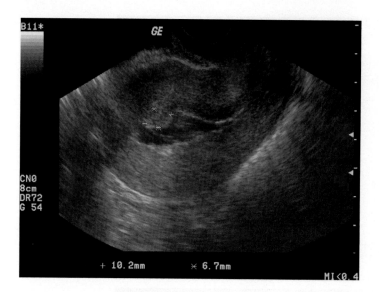

Fig. 7. Saline infusion sonohysterogram of a perimenopausal patient who had abnormal uterine bleeding. A polypoid lesion is seen extending near the anterior fundal region. This lesion measures 10.2 × 6.7 (*calipers*). At the time of dilation and curettage and hysteroscopy, a polyp was identified that was confirmed by pathology.

Inadequate distension of the cavity

In some patients, a patulous cervix results in a great deal of fluid running out transcervically. Other patients have fluid going out through fallopian tubes, even with slow injection and minimal pressure. As in hysteroscopy, some cavities are more difficult to distend than others. The clinician should check the position of the catheter, looking for its acoustic shadow most of the way to the uterine fundus. Unlike hysteroscopy (which requires distension for visualization), however, this procedure requires very little fluid to outline the cavity. Even a small ribbon of fluid acts as a sufficient interface to distinguish anterior and posterior endometrial surfaces and to outline endometrial pathology.

Summary

Abnormal uterine bleeding, whether it occurs in peri- or postmenopausal patients, is an important clinical concern and accounts for much medical intervention. When bleeding occurs in women older than 40 years (and in any postmenopausal woman), endometrial "assessment" is mandatory. In the past and even currently, many clinicians prefer to begin such assessment with blind endometrial sampling. This article presents an ultrasound-based approach to such patients. When present, a thin, distinct endometrial echo excludes significant pathology, assuming it is performed at an appropriate time if the patient is cycling. If a thin, distinct endometrial echo is not visualized (inadequate visualization or presence of thickened echo),

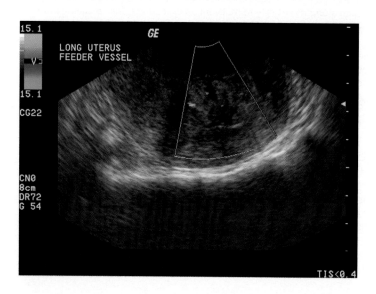

Fig. 8. Long-axis view of the uterus in a patient who had abnormal uterine bleeding. Color flow Doppler imaging clearly identifies a central feeder vessel. Presence of such a feeder vessel can be used to make the diagnosis of polyp even in the absence of saline infusion.

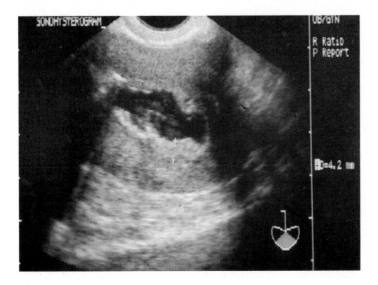

Fig. 9. Transvaginal pelvic scan of a patient 19 days since her last episode of bleeding. The endometrial surface is irregular. The irregular surface is not unusual, especially in patients who have had previous dilation and curettage procedures, myomectomies, childbirth, and so forth. The irregular surface to the endometrium, here identified as "moguls," can be misleading. Performing the procedure this long after the last bleeding episode can be fraught with error and should be avoided.

then saline infusion sonohysterography can help to triage patients to (1) no anatomic pathology, (2) globally thickened anatomic pathology that may be evaluated with blind endometrial sampling, or (3) focal abnormalities that must be evaluated under direct vision. Such an ultrasound-based approach not only helps to exclude endometrial carcinoma but also identifies the source of any bleeding for better clinical management.

References

[1] Awwad JT, Toth TL, Schiff I. Abnormal uterine bleeding in the perimenopause. Int J fertile 1993;38:261–9.

[2] SEER Cancer Statistics Review, 1873–1996 [serial online]. Available at: http://seer.cancer.gov/csr/1973_1996/index.html. Accessed August 26, 2005.

[3] Iatrakis G, Diakakis I, Kourounis G, et al. Postmenopausal uterine bleeding. Clin Exp Obstet Gynecol 1997;24:157.

[4] ACOG practice bulletin: management of anovulatory bleeding. ACOG Committee on Practice Bulletins–Gynecology. American College of Obstetricians and Gynecologists. Int J Gynaecol Obstet 2001;72:263–71.

[5] Ricci JV. Gynaecologic surgery and instruments of the nineteenth century prior to the antiseptic age. In: Ricci JV, editor. The development of gynaecological surgery and instruments. Philadelphia: Blakiston; 1949. p. 326–8.

[6] Word B, Gravlee LC, Widemon GL. The fallacy of simple uterine curettage. Obstet Gynecol 1958;12:642–5.

[7] Vuopala S. Diagnostic accuracy and clinical applicability of cytological and histological methods for investigating endometrial carcinoma. Acta Obstet Gyneocl Scand Suppl 1977;70:1–72.

[8] Kaunitz AM, Masciello AS, Ostrowsky M, et al. Comparison of endometrial Pipelle and Vabra aspirator. J Reprod Med 1988;33:427–31.

[9] Rodriguez MJ, Platt LD, Medearis AL, et al. The use of transvaginal sonography for evaluation of postmenopausal size and morphology. Am J Obstet Gynecol 1988;159:810–4.

[10] Stovall TG, Photopulos GJ, Poston WM, et al. Pipelle endometrial sampling in patients with known endometrial cancer. Obstet Gynecol 1991;77:954–6.

[11] Guido RS, Kanbour A, Ruhn M, et al. Pipelle endometrial sampling sensitivity in the detection of endometrial cancer. J Reprod Med 1995;40:553–5.

[12] Goldstein SR. Endovaginal ultrasound. 2nd edition. New York: Wiley Liss; 1991.

[13] Goldstein SR, Nachtigall M, Snyder JR, et al. Endometrial assessment by vaginal ultrasonography before endometrial sampling in patients with postmenopausal bleeding. Am J Obstet Gynecol 1990;163:119–23.

[14] Granberg S, Wikland M, Karlsson B, et al. Endometrial thickness as measured by endovaginal ultrasound ultrasonography for identifying endometrial abnormality. Am J Obstet Gynecol 1991;164:47–52.

[15] Goldstein RB, Bree RL, Benson CB, et al. Evaluation of the woman with postmenopausal bleeding: Society of Radiologists in Ultrasound–Sponsored Consensus Conference statement. J Ultrasound Med 2001;20:1025–36.

[16] Goldstein SR. Postmenopausal endometrial fluid collections revisited: look at the doughnut rather than the hole. Obstet Gynecol 1994;83:738–40.

[17] Randolph JR, Ying YK, Maier DB, et al. Comparison of realtime ultrasonography, hysterosalpingography, and laparoscopy/hysteroscopy in evaluation of uterine abnormalities and tubal patency. Fertil Steril 1986;46:828–32.

[18] Parsons AK, Lense JJ. Sonohysterography for endometrial abnormalities: preliminary results. J Clin Ultrasound 1993;21:87–95.

[19] Syrop C, Sahakian V. Transvaginal sonographic detection of endometrial polyps with fluid contrast augmentation. Obstet Gynecol 1992;79:1041–3.

[20] Goldstein SR. Use of ultrasonohysterography for triage of perimenopausal patients with unexplained uterine bleeding. Am J Obstet Gynecol 1994;170:565–70.

[21] Goldstein SR, Zelzter I, Horan CK, et al. Ultrasonography-based triage for perimenopausal patients with abnormal uterine bleeding. Am J Obstet Gynecol 1997;177:102–8.

[22] Dijkhuzien FPHLJ, Brolmann HAM, Potters AE, et al. The accuracy of transvaginal ultrasonography in the diagnosis of endometrial abnormalities. Obstet Gynecol 1996;87:345–9.

[23] Timmerman D, Verguts J, Konstantinovic ML, et al. The pedicle artery sign based on sonography with color Doppler imaging can replace second-stage tests in women with abnormal vaginal bleeding. Ultrasound Obstet Gynecol 2003;22:166–71.

[24] Wolman I, Groutz A, Gordon D, et al. Timing of sonohysterography in menstruating women. Gynecol Obstet Invest 1999;48:254–8.

[25] Dessole S, Farina M, Rubattu G, et al. Side effects and complications of sonhystyerosalpingography. Fertil Steril 2003;80:620–4.

[26] Cooper JM, Brady RM. Intraoperative and early postoperative complications of operative hysteroscopy. Obstet Gynecol Clin North Am 2000;27:347–66.

[27] Tuveng JM, Vold I, Jerve F, et al. Hysterosalpingography: value in estimating tubal function, and risk of infectious complications. Acta Eur Fertl 1985;16:125–8.

[28] DeVore GR, Schwartz PE, Morris J. Hysterography: a 5-year follow-up in patients with endometrial carcinoma. Obstet Gynecol 1982;60:369–72.

[29] Alcazar JL, Errasti R, Zornoza A. Saline infusion sonohysterography in endometrial cancer: assessment of malignant cells dissemination risk. Acta Obstet Gynecol Scand 2000;79:321–2.

ELSEVIER
SAUNDERS

RADIOLOGIC
CLINICS
OF NORTH AMERICA

Radiol Clin N Am 44 (2006) 911–923

Sonographic Evaluation of the Child with Lower Abdominal or Pelvic Pain

Peter J. Strouse, MD

- General approach
- Gastrointestinal disorders
- Appendicitis
- Mesenteric adenitis
- Intussusception
- Duplication cyst
- Inflammatory bowel disease
- Henoch-Schönlein purpura
- Meckel diverticulum
- Small bowel obstruction
- Omental infarction
- Urinary tract disorders

Renal stone
Urinary tract infection
Infected urachus
- Gynecologic disorders
Hematometrocolpos/hematocolpos
Cyst/ruptured cyst
Ovarian neoplasms
Ectopic pregnancy
Tubo-ovarian abscess
Ovarian torsion
- Summary
- References

At many centers, CT has become the primary imaging modality for children who have abdominal pain. CT, however, delivers a substantial radiation dose, which is of particular concern in the pediatric patient. In contrast, sonography does not expose the patient to ionizing radiation. Properly performed, sonography is capable of providing useful diagnostic information in the child who has lower abdominal or pelvic pain. In many children and with many disorders, sonography proves to be the only imaging modality that may be required. In this article, the usefulness of sonography in evaluating disorders producing lower abdominal or pelvic pain in a child is reviewed.

General approach

Work-up of the child who has lower abdominal or pelvic pain begins with a careful history and physical examination. Pertinent laboratory examination may be helpful. The decision of whether to image and which modality to use is guided by information obtained from the history, physical examination, and basic laboratory examination.

Abdominal pain is a common complaint in children. It is one of the most common reasons for an unscheduled visit to the pediatrician's office or a visit to an emergency department. The overwhelming majority of children presenting with abdominal pain do not have an organic condition requiring medical or surgical intervention [1,2]. Findings that suggest there is an organic etiology to the patient's complaints of pain are pain that is not periumbilical or pain that migrates from a periumbilical location, fever, leukocytosis, abnormal urinalysis, blood in stool, or a palpable mass. When one of these findings is present, further evaluation with imaging is likely required.

This article was originally published in *Ultrasound Clinics* 1:3, July 2006.
Section of Pediatric Radiology, C.S. Mott Children's Hospital, Room F3503, Department of Radiology, University of Michigan Health System, 1500 East Medical Center Drive, Ann Arbor, MI 48103-0252, USA
E-mail address: pstrouse@umich.edu

Imaging protocols naturally vary from institution to institution and even between different physician users and imaging providers within the same institution. If pathology of the female pelvis is suspected, ultrasound is firmly indicated as an initial imaging step. With suspected gastrointestinal pathology, radiography, sonography, or CT may be used, depending on the suspected disorder, the age of the child, and institutional preferences. This is also true for suspected urinary tract pathology. When there is uncertainty of the origin of a child's pain, preliminary examination with sonography is a good first step, because it does not expose the child to ionizing radiation and it guides the proper use of other imaging studies.

Gastrointestinal disorders

Regardless of the disorder being imaged, evaluation of the gastrointestinal tract with sonography requires meticulous technique. Air is the enemy of the ultrasound beam. Graded compression of the abdomen is required to obliterate and displace gas from bowel in the field of view. Although tensely distended gas filled bowel or guarding by the patient may occasionally obscure visualization, careful, gradual compression usually achieves visualization of deeper structures. Visualization of bowel is improved by use of a linear array transducer. Compression also serves to bring the pathologic bowel in the focal zone ("sweet spot") of the transducer.

Well-trained sonographic technologists may be skilled in performing ultrasound of the gastrointestinal tract; however, the value of witnessing scanning of the patient or, better yet, scanning the patient oneself, cannot be overstated. The realtime capability of sonography allows for a directed scan ("show me where it hurts"). The reaction of the patient to palpation with the transducer also yields information. The suspicion of underlying pathology may be heightened or lessened by observing or performing this limited physical examination.

Appendicitis

Appendicitis is overwhelmingly the most common surgical cause for abdominal pain in childhood. Nonetheless, only a small percentage of children presenting with abdominal pain prove to have appendicitis [1–3]. Clinical findings suggestive of appendicitis include periumbilical pain migrating to the right lower quadrant, fever, and leukocytosis. Until the late 1980s the diagnosis of appendicitis was purely clinical. Unfortunately, clinical evaluation of appendicitis is imprecise. Historically, an accepted 15% to 20% negative appendectomy rate was balanced against a desire to limit complications caused by perforation of undiagnosed appendicitis.

Graded compression ultrasound for the evaluation of appendicitis was introduced by Puylaert in 1986 [4]. As previously described, a linear array transducer is used. Compression is applied gradually so as to be better tolerated by the patient. The examination is best started by asking the patient, "Where does it hurt?" (Do *not* tell the patient to "point to where it hurts.") The patient who has uncomplicated appendicitis often points to a specific location. The indicated area of the abdomen is the starting point for scanning. It is striking how often the abnormal appendix is found immediately beneath the site where the patient indicates the pain. If the appendix is not immediately identified, a systematic search of the right lower quadrant and pelvis is performed. Careful sweeps in the longitudinal and transverse planes are performed. Less experienced sonographers frequently make the mistake of not providing adequate compression. With adequate compression, the posterior abdominal wall, the psoas muscle, and the iliac vasculature are seen (Fig. 1). Illustrations in Puylaert's original article nicely demonstrate the degree of compression required [4].

Some investigators have indicated a high rate of identifying the normal appendix [5,6]. To exclude appendicitis, the bulbous tip of the appendix must be seen. Identification of the normal appendix is the best evidence that the patient does not have appendicitis. Identification of the normal appendix, however, is extremely difficult and time consuming.

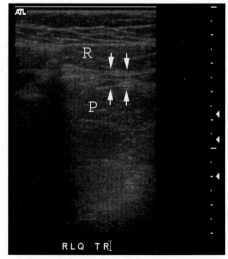

Fig. 1. A 15-year-old girl who had a normal right lower quadrant ultrasound. Adequate compression is indicated by visualization of the posterior abdominal wall, including the psoas muscle (P). Note the short distance (*between the pairs of arrows*) between the rectus abdominus muscle (R) in the anterior abdominal wall and psoas muscle posteriorly.

In most practices and for most patients the normal appendix is never seen. Lack of identification of an abnormal appendix is good evidence against the diagnosis of the appendicitis; however, some uncertainty inevitably persists as to whether an inflamed appendix may have been missed. This uncertainty may be heightened or tempered by witnessing the patient's reaction to being scanned. If the patient is completely comfortable with deep palpation by the transducer, he or she is unlikely to have appendicitis. If the patient is very uncomfortable to minimal compression with the transducer, the likelihood of underlying pathology is higher.

The normal appendix is 6 mm or less in diameter and compressible (Fig. 2). The abnormal appendix is 7 mm or greater in diameter and noncompressible (Fig. 3) [4,5]. The appendix is tubular and blind ending. An appendicolith may or may not be present (Fig. 4). If the appendix is truly abnormal, it should be re-demonstrable—one should be able to verify the abnormality by removing the transducer, replacing it, and re-finding the abnormality. Color Doppler may show increased flow indicating inflammation [7]. In the setting of perforation, the appendix may no longer be visible [8–10]. A mass or abscess may be found [5,8]. Such findings are nonspecific; however, as appendicitis is the most likely diagnosis in this setting, perforated appendicitis should be suspected [9].

In experienced hands, ultrasound performs well in the diagnosis of appendicitis [4,11,12]. Although CT is probably more sensitive and more specific, it is only slightly better than ultrasound. Disadvantages of ultrasound include dependence on the operator and lack of a global view of the abdomen and pelvis [13]. Both of these disadvantages are surmounted by CT. In most head-to-head comparisons, CT exceeds sonography in sensitivity and specificity [13–16]. At most institutions in the United States, CT has thus supplanted ultrasound as the chief diagnostic modality in the diagnosis of appendicitis. This is somewhat unfortunate given the radiation exposure associated with CT and the increasing reliance on imaging for diagnosis, leading to more children with lesser symptoms or suspicion for disease being imaged.

What is the proper role of ultrasound in suspected appendicitis? Before answering this question, it is important to acknowledge that there are two questions asked of us by our surgical colleagues: "Does this child have appendicitis?" And, "Is it perforated?" At many institutions, surgical management of perforated and nonperforated appendicitis differs. In an ideal setting ultrasound serves as a screening examination for appendicitis [12,15,17,18]. Most children who have appendicitis would be diagnosed using sonography, thus avoiding a CT. In cases in which there was a high clinical suspicion or equivocal sonographic findings, CT would be performed. In cases in which perforated appendicitis is strongly suspected, imaging could commence directly with CT. This model has worked well at some pediatric institutions [17,19,20]; however, when one imaging study exceeds another in accuracy (as viewed by our clinical colleagues) it becomes difficult to supplant in clinical work. It is incumbent on radiologists to maintain the skills of appendiceal sonography to provide a radiation-free imaging alternative to CT.

Mesenteric adenitis

The diagnosis of mesenteric adenitis is one of exclusion. This is not a diagnosis that is accepted by all.

A
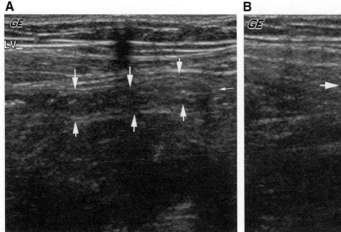
B
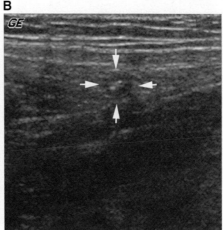

Fig. 2. An 11-year-old girl who had a normal appendix (*arrows*) seen on (*A*) longitudinal and (*B*) transverse views. This appendix is 4 mm in diameter. *Small arrow*, tip of the appendix.

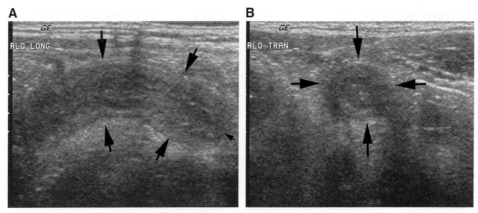

Fig. 3. A 5-year-old boy who had nonperforated appendicitis. An enlarged appendix (*arrows*) measuring 12 mm in diameter is seen on (*A*) longitudinal and (*B*) transverse views. *Small arrow*, tip of the appendix.

Children may be assigned the diagnosis of mesenteric adenitis when enlarged lymph nodes are seen in the right lower quadrant in the absence of other pathology (Fig. 5). Mildly prominent right lower quadrant mesenteric lymph nodes are a normal finding in children, and criteria for what constitutes abnormal enlargement are not well defined [21,22]. Enlarged lymph nodes may also be seen with various pathologies, including appendicitis, inflammatory bowel disease, yersinia ileitis, and Henoch-Schönlein purpura [23]. The diagnosis of mesenteric adenitis is not used at the author's institution.

Intussusception

At many institutions, including the author's, ultrasound has become the chief diagnostic method of

confirming the presence of intussusception [24,25]. Improvement of ultrasound equipment has allowed for this development. Concomitantly, an unacceptably high and increasing negative rate for enemas performed for suspected intussusception has prompted the development of new imaging algorithms to avoid numerous unnecessary enema examinations in young children [24,25].

Ultrasound performs well in identifying ileocolic intussusceptions [24–28]. False negatives are rare. Intussusceptions are seen as large masses, usually approximately 4 cm in diameter or greater. The longitudinal dimension of the mass varies depending on the length of the intussusception. Most intussusceptions are encountered in the right midabdomen or subhepatic space; however, the mass can be found anywhere within the abdomen or pelvis. The sonographic search therefore begins in the right midabdomen, but must include the whole abdomen if no intussusception is encountered on the right. In the author's experience, a negative

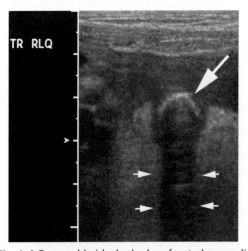

Fig. 4. A 5-year-old girl who had perforated appendicitis. An appendicolith (*large arrow*) is seen with a posterior acoustic shadow (*small arrows*). A layer of soft tissue around the appendicolith is appendiceal wall. The appendix was not seen otherwise.

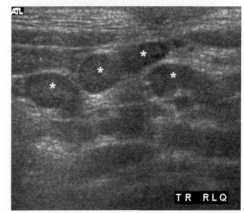

Fig. 5. A 3-year-old boy who had mildly enlarged right lower quadrant lymph nodes (*asterisks*).

ultrasound is highly predictive of the absence of an intussusception. Rarely, if clinical suspicion persists, an enema still may be performed.

On ultrasound, an ileocolic intussusception is seen as a large mass with a layered appearance or a thick hypoechoic outer wall caused by edematous bowel wall (Fig. 6) [24–29]. The center of the lesion is hyperechoic owing to mesenteric fat within the intussusception. Lymph nodes are often present within the hyperechoic center (Fig. 7) [29,30]. These are seen as small oval hypoechoic structures, usually less than 1 cm. There are no sonographic findings that preclude subsequent enema for treatment; however, some findings have been identified that may indicate a lesser likelihood of successful reduction and a higher likelihood of complicating perforation. These findings include lack of blood flow within the intussusception on Doppler evaluation and trapped fluid within layers on the intussusception [29,31,32].

Other disorders may be mistaken for an ileocolic intussusception. Small bowel intussusceptions appear similar but are smaller in diameter and often transient (Fig. 8) [33]. Disorders that cause bowel wall thickening may appear similar, including inflammatory bowel disease, lymphoma, and intramural hemorrhage.

Ultrasound may also demonstrate findings suggestive of a lead point of an intussusception [34]. Only 5% of pediatric patients have a lead point. Lead points that may be demonstrated by sonography include a duplication cyst or bowel wall thickening caused by inflammation or intramural

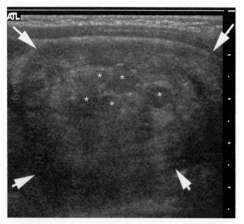

Fig. 7. A 3-year-old boy who had intussusception (*arrows*). Multiple lymph nodes (*asterisks*) are seen within mesenteric fat within the intussusception.

hemorrhage as may be seen with Henoch-Schönlein purpura.

Ultrasound has been used at some institutions to monitor reduction of intussusception with saline, water, and even air enemas [35,36]. This further spares the patient radiation exposure. A disadvantage of the technique is a limited field of view during the reduction. This technique has had very limited use in the United States.

Duplication cyst

Classic duplication cysts have a characteristic appearance on ultrasound of the double layered wall (Fig. 9) [37,38]. The inner layer is hyperechoic mucosa and the outer layer is hypoechoic muscle. Unfortunately with inflammation, the layers may be

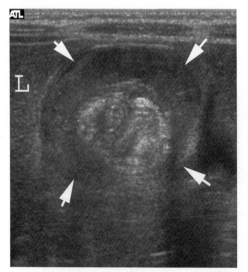

Fig. 6. A 4-month-old boy who had intussusception (*arrows*). A thick hypoechoic "donut" is seen with echogenic mesenteric fat centrally within the mass. L, liver.

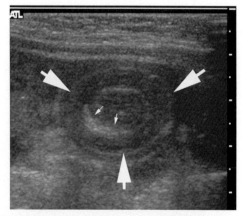

Fig. 8. A 3-year-old boy who had distal small bowel intussusception caused by Henoch-Schönlein purpura. The intussusception (*large arrows*) is less than 2 cm in diameter, much smaller than the typical ileocolic intussusception. *Small arrows*, mesenteric fat within the intussusception.

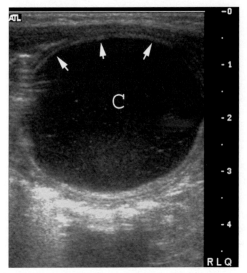

Fig. 9. An infant girl presenting with small bowel obstruction secondary to volvulus around an enteric duplication cyst. This cyst (C) measures 3.5 cm in diameter. Portions of the cyst wall show the characteristic double-layered appearance with echogenic mucosa internally (*arrows*) and hypoechoic muscle externally.

present within the cyst, it may secrete enzymes, leading to inflammation and presentation with pain.

Differential considerations for a fluid-filled cystic mass in the lower abdomen include omental or mesenteric cysts and ovarian neoplasm. Omental and mesenteric cysts are usually asymptomatic unto themselves, unless there is an associated obstruction or torsion of bowel.

Inflammatory bowel disease

Inflammatory bowel disease produces bowel wall thickening [41]. If a segment of small bowel or colon with a thick wall is identified by sonography, the diagnosis should be suspected. Differentiation of abnormal small bowel from abnormal colon may be difficult, but may be inferred by anatomic location. Correlation with clinical presentation is helpful. The inflamed small bowel of Crohn disease is typically on the order of 3 cm in diameter, substantially larger than the typical inflamed appendix. In transverse, the appearance is similar to an intussusception; however, in longitudinal views the abnormal bowel is more elongate and does not have the overlapped or invaginated appearance of an intussusception (Fig. 10). Hyperemia is evident on Doppler interrogation. Occasionally hypertrophied adipose tissue is seen adjacent to the inflamed loop of bowel. This tissue appears homogeneously hyperechoic.

At some centers, mostly in Europe, sonography has been used to longitudinally monitor Crohn disease activity [41,42].

Other infectious or inflammatory bowel diseases may appear similar to Crohn disease, including

obscured, lessening the specificity [39]. Nonetheless, demonstration of a cystic mass adjacent to bowel should prompt consideration of a duplication cyst.

Duplication cysts are congenital malformations of bowel that can occur anywhere in the gastrointestinal tract [38,40]. The most common locations are at the esophagus followed by terminal ileum [40]. Classically, children present early in childhood as the cyst distends with fluid. If gastric mucosa is

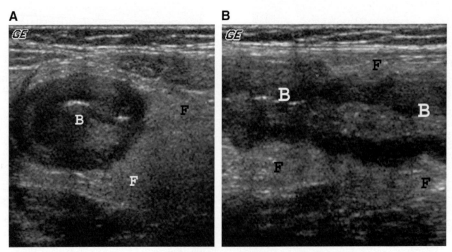

Fig. 10. A 9-year-old girl who had acute abdominal pain as the presenting manifestation of Crohn disease. (*A*) Transverse and (*B*) longitudinal images show an abnormal segment of small bowel (B) with prominent echogenic mucosa centrally and a markedly thickened wall. Note prominent adjacent fat (F).

ulcerative colitis, pseudomembranous colitis, yersinia ileitis, and infectious entero-colitides. In a neutropenic patient, marked thickening of the cecal and proximal ascending colon wall may indicate typhlitis (neutropenic colitis). Correlation with clinical history and physical examination may help differentiate inflammatory disorders causing bowel wall thickening.

Henoch-Schönlein purpura

Henoch-Schönlein purpura (HSP) is an idiopathic vasculitis. Although the disorder may involve several organ systems, the chief sources of morbidity are involvement of the gastrointestinal and genitourinary tract [43]. These children develop a characteristic purpuric rash; however, involvement of the gastrointestinal tract may precede development of the rash.

In children who have HSP, the bowel wall is thickened by inflammation and intramural hemorrhage (Fig. 11) [43–45]. Bowel wall abnormality is often discontinuous. Increased flow is seen on Doppler interrogation. Free intraperitoneal fluid and mild mesenteric lymph node enlargement are common findings. The mural abnormality of HSP may act as a lead point for an intussusception (see Fig. 8) [43,44]. If the patient has not yet been diagnosed with HSP, the finding of bowel wall thickening, with or without an intussusception, should prompt consideration of the diagnosis.

Meckel diverticulum

Meckel diverticulum is a remnant of the omphalomesenteric duct [46]. Meckel diverticulum can present in various ways. In addition to the classic presentation with painless gastrointestinal hemorrhage, Meckel diverticulum can present with inflammation (Meckel diverticulitis), as a lead point for an intussusception, or as the focal point of a small bowel volvulus (usually in association with an omphalomesenteric band) [26,46].

Meckel diverticulum is rarely diagnosed prospectively; however, sonography may identify the inflamed diverticulum, an intussusception, or a small bowel obstruction caused by a Meckel diverticulum [26,46]. Identification of the appendix as separate from the area of inflammation, location to the left of midline, and larger size than is typical for an inflamed appendix all suggest Meckel diverticulitis as opposed to appendicitis [46,47].

Small bowel obstruction

Children who have small bowel obstruction are often evaluated with means other than ultrasound,

because the history and physical examination findings lead the clinician to suspect the presence of an obstruction. Many of the previously discussed entities may cause a small bowel obstruction. The presence of fluid-filled dilated loops on sonography may suggest an obstruction, particularly if a caliber change is demonstrated and collapsed loops are seen further distal. Sonography may be helpful in demonstrating the cause of an obstruction (Fig. 12) [48].

Omental infarction

Omental infarction is usually caused by torsion of an omental appendage. The cause for torsion and infarction is unknown. In some patients the onset of symptoms has been linked to a large meal. Patients present with sudden onset pain. Patients are usually but not invariably afebrile and without elevation of the white blood cell count. The clinical presentation may mimic appendicitis.

Although the diagnosis is more readily made by CT, sonography can also make the diagnosis, particularly when the operator is familiar with the entity and searches for the findings. On ultrasound, the infarcted omentum is seen as a lenticular or ovoid mass immediately behind the anterior abdominal wall, usually in the right lower quadrant [49,50]. The mass is homogeneous and hyperechoic and corresponds with the patient's point of maximal tenderness.

Omental infarction is a self-limited condition. Surgery is not required. Making the diagnosis may spare the patient an unnecessary surgery.

Urinary tract disorders

Renal stone

Renal colic is in the differential diagnosis for lower abdominal pain in children. Pain is usually referred to the flank, but may present in the lower abdomen or pelvis. Renal calculi are much less common in children than in adults; however, they are not infrequently encountered [51]. Use of CT for the diagnosis of renal calculi has become commonplace even in children; however, the radiation dose associated with CT must be considered [52]. At initial presentation with a calculus, the diagnosis may not initially be entertained and ultrasound may be performed. In a child who has a history of calculi, performance of repeated renal stone protocol CT studies is to be discouraged, particularly if the clinical presentation is consistent with a recurrent calculus. Ultrasound can be useful in these children to evaluate for collecting system dilatation, which together with the clinical presentation offers confirmatory evidence of the presence of an obstructing

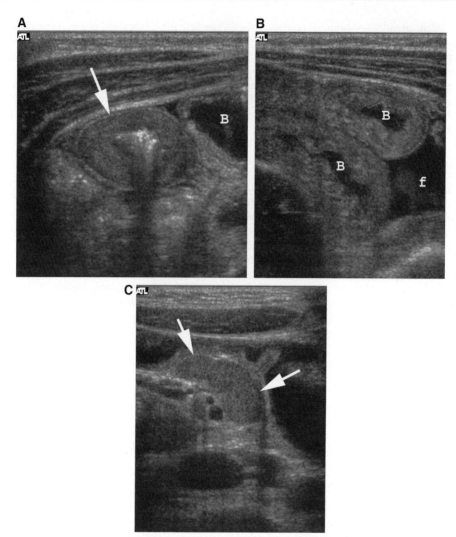

Fig. 11. A 6-year-old girl presenting with abdominal pain caused by Henoch-Schönlein purpura. (*A*) An involved bowel loop (*arrow*) with a thick wall is seen adjacent to a normal bowel loop (B). (*B*) Additional thick-walled bowel loops seen in longitudinal view. F, free fluid. (*C*) Mildly enlarged lymph nodes (*arrows*).

calculus [53]. Occasionally sonography may demonstrate an impacted distal ureteral calculus (Fig. 13).

Urinary tract infection

Children who have cystitis caused by lower urinary tract infection or other causes may present with pelvic pain. Sonography may show thickening of the urinary bladder wall. Unfortunately, thickening of the bladder wall is difficult to interpret. The wall of an underdistended bladder may appear very thick. Thickening disproportionate to the degree of distension, irregularity, and asymmetry of thickening are features that suggest pathologic bladder wall thickening as opposed to spurious thickening from underdistention.

Upper urinary tract infections usually present flank pain higher in the abdomen, as do other disorders of the kidney.

Infected urachus

Infected urachus is a rare cause of lower abdominal pain. The urachus is an embryonic connection from the anterior aspect of the dome of the bladder to the umbilicus [54]. The urachus may persist in its entirety (patent urachus) or either end (urachal sinus, urachal diverticulum). If the midportion persists with both ends obliterated, the patient may develop a urachal cyst. These cysts are often asymptomatic until they become superinfected. On sonography, a complex, cystic mass is identified at the midline

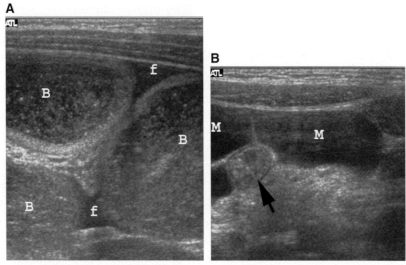

Fig. 12. A 3-year-old boy who had small bowel obstruction caused by focal volvulus related to a mesenteric cyst. (*A*) Dilated small bowel loops (B) containing fecal material, consistent with a small bowel obstruction. F, free fluid. (*B*) The mesenteric cyst (M) is seen as a septated, fluid-filled mass. Note that it partially encases a normal caliber bowel loop (*arrow*).

between umbilicus and bladder [54], and there may be surrounding inflammation.

Gynecologic disorders

Hematometrocolpos/hematocolpos

Hematometrocolpos presenting in adolescent girls is usually secondary to vaginal obstruction by an imperforate hymen. The patient presents at puberty with primary amenorrhea and cyclic lower abdominal or pelvic pain. Ultrasound shows a fluid-filled mass posterior to the bladder representing the dilated vagina. The uterus may (hematometrocolpos) or may not (hematocolpos) be dilated also. The dilated uterus can be differentiated from the vagina by the cervical margin and thicker wall. Occasionally the fallopian tubes may be dilated.

Hematometros and hematometrocolpos may also occur because of congenital uterine and vaginal anomalies presenting at the time of puberty, caused by obstruction and distension in response to the onset of menses [55]. Not infrequently in such patients, a duplication is present with obstruction of one side.

Cyst/ruptured cyst

A ruptured functional cyst or corpus luteum cyst is a common cause of pelvic pain in teenage girls [56]. Usually the causal cyst is no longer evident because it has decompressed itself through rupture. Sometimes a hyperechoic or complex cystic mass of the ovary persists. A variable amount of free fluid is present within the pelvis. Debris from hemorrhage may be present within the fluid.

Ovarian or paraovarian cysts may cause pain in themselves. Ovarian cysts in adolescent girls are usually functional cysts, forming in response to the cycling hormones of the menstrual cycle. Given the low incidence of malignant ovarian tumors, it is usually sufficient to obtain a follow-up sonogram after at least one full menstrual cycle to confirm resolution of the finding.

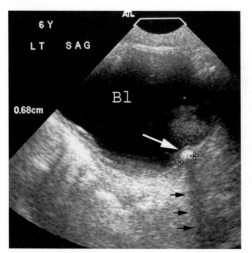

Fig. 13. A 6-year-old girl who had impacted distal ureteral calculus (*large arrow*). A posterior acoustic shadow (*small arrows*) is seen. Bl, bladder.

Ovarian neoplasms

Ovarian neoplasms in children are usually benign [57,58]. Most tumors present as a painless mass;

however, some tumors present with pelvic pain, particularly if the tumor is acting as a nidus for torsion. As discussed previously, functional cysts are the most common cause of an ovarian mass [56,57]. Persistence of the cyst on follow-up examination, continued symptoms, or identification of any solid component within the mass are all features that may suggest neoplasm.

Ectopic pregnancy

In the sexually active teenage girl, ectopic pregnancy is an important consideration in the differential diagnosis of pelvic pain [59]. Ectopic pregnancy can be life threatening because of hemorrhage. If a patient who has pelvic pain has been sexually active, a pregnancy test is warranted. If the pregnancy test is positive and no intrauterine pregnancy is found, ectopic pregnancy must be strongly considered until proven otherwise. The differential diagnosis for a positive pregnancy test without demonstration of an intrauterine gestation is early intrauterine pregnancy, spontaneous abortion, or ectopic pregnancy. Serial serum β-HCG levels and serial sonography may help to differentiate these possibilities.

Sonography may demonstrate a living ectopic pregnancy outside of the uterus. A gestational sac may be seen in the adnexa (Fig. 14). Findings of adnexal mass and free fluid are nonspecific, but in the setting of a positive pregnancy test and lack of a demonstrable intrauterine pregnancy, these findings are suggestive of an ectopic pregnancy [60,61]. Endovaginal scanning is preferred when evaluating for early pregnancy and possible ectopic pregnancy [62].

Tubo-ovarian abscess

Unfortunately pelvic inflammatory disease and tubo-ovarian abscess are also not infrequent diagnoses in the sexually active teenager [63,64]. In a sexually active teenage girl, gynecologic infection should be in the differential diagnosis for lower abdominal or pelvic pain. A good history and physical examination, including a pelvic examination, may suggest the correct diagnosis. The clinical presentation and physical examination findings overlap with appendicitis, particularly when the pathology is on the right. Sonography is the study of choice in these patients. It demonstrates abnormalities related to the gynecologic tract, and graded compression examination of the right lower quadrant can be performed during the same examination to assess for appendicitis.

In the absence of tubal obstruction, sonographic findings with pelvic inflammatory disease may be normal. Pelvic inflammation may blur margins of the uterus. Free fluid may be present but is nonspecific. Fluid-filled adnexal tubular structures or complex cystic masses in the presence of clinical findings suggesting infection should raise concern for tubo-ovarian abscess (Fig. 15) [64].

Ovarian torsion

Ovarian torsion may occur in a child of any age, but is most common in the neonate and in the adolescent. Increased incidence of ovarian torsion in neonates may relate to enlargement of the ovaries related to stimulation from maternal hormones. The incidence increases again at adolescence in response to hormonal changes. Although underlying masses may act as a nidus for torsion and do

A
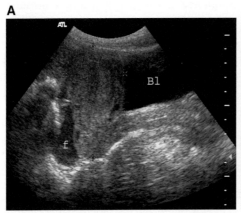

B
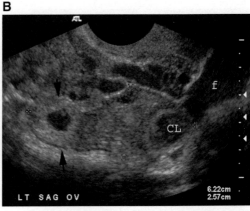

Fig. 14. A teenage girl who had an ectopic pregnancy. The patient was 9 weeks from her last period, had a β-HCG level of 3370 mIU/mL, and presented with acute left pelvic pain. (*A*) Transabdominal images show an empty uterine cavity and free fluid (F). Cursors delimit the uterus. Bl, bladder. Absence of intrauterine pregnancy was confirmed by endovaginal scanning. (*B*) Endovaginal image of the left adnexa. An ectopic tubal ring (*arrows*) is identified adjacent to the left ovary (*cursors*). A corpus luteum is seen within the ovary (CL). F, free fluid. (Images courtesy of Alexis V. Nees, MD, Ann Arbor, Michigan).

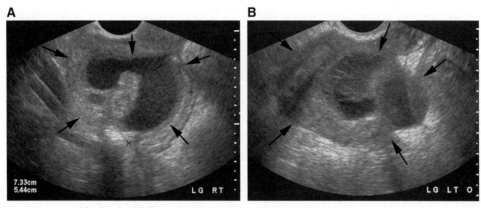

A   **B**

Fig. 15. A teenage girl who had bilateral tubo-ovarian abscesses. Complex, cystic, and solid adnexal masses (*arrows*) are seen on the (*A*) right and (*B*) left. (Images courtesy of Alexis V. Nees, MD, Ann Arbor, Michigan).

increase the risk for torsion, most torsed ovaries in children do not bear an underlying lesion. It is believed that abnormal fixation of the ovary may predispose these ovaries to torsion.

Patients who have ovarian torsion present with sudden onset pelvic or lower abdominal pain. There is often a history of similar episodes of pain before presentation. The patient may have a slight fever and borderline elevation of the white blood cell count, often confounding the clinical diagnosis. On physical examination, a tender mass may be felt.

If there is an underlying mass, it is well shown by sonography. A torsed ovary with a cyst may mimic a gastrointestinal duplication in appearance, occasionally showing a double-layered wall [65]. In torsed ovaries without an underlying mass, the ovary itself appears as a mass because of swelling. The sonographic appearance of the torsed ovary varies from completely solid to cystic, with most having a predominantly solid or mixed solid and cystic appearance [66,67]. The only gray scale finding considered specific for ovarian torsion is a solid mass with small cysts (follicles) at its periphery (Fig. 16). The torsed ovary usually sits in the

cul de sac behind the uterus or unusually anterior. Normal ovary is not seen at the expected adnexal location. The value of Doppler interrogation of the torsed ovary is somewhat limited [67]. In the prepubertal ovary, flow may be difficult to demonstrate in a normal ovary, making it difficult to determine if flow is absent. The ovary has dual blood supply from the ovarian and uterine arteries. Flow thus may be present even in the presence of torsion. Nonetheless, if flow is not demonstrable within an enlarged ovary and flow is demonstrable within the contralateral normal ovary, torsion should be suspected.

The CT findings of torsion are less specific; however, CT may also demonstrate peripheral follicles within a torsed ovary. Sonography may be helpful in confirming the diagnosis when CT findings are equivocal.

Summary

Sonography is an excellent modality for the evaluation of the child who has lower abdominal or pelvicpain. Whether or not a specific diagnosis (ie, appendicitis) is suspected, versatility and lack of ionizing radiation make sonography an excellent first line of imaging.

References

[1] Buchert GS. Abdominal pain in children: an emergency practitioner's guide. Emerg Med Clin North Am 1989;7:497–517.

[2] Scholer SJ, Pituch K, Orr DP, et al. Clinical outcomes of children with acute abdominal pain. Pediatrics 1996;98:680–5.

[3] Reynolds SL, Jaffe DM. Diagnosing abdominal pain in a pediatric emergency department. Pediatr Emerg Care 1992;8:126–8.

[4] Puylaert JB. Acute appendicitis: US evaluation using graded compression. Radiology 1986;158: 355–60.

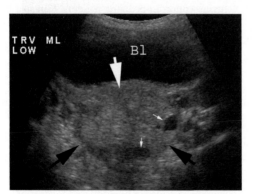

Fig. 16. A 2-year-old girl who had a torsed ovary (*large arrows*). A solid mass is seen posterior to the bladder (*Bl*). Note some peripheral follicles (*small arrows*).

[5] Sivit CJ. Diagnosis of acute appendicitis in children: spectrum of sonographic findings. Am J Roentgenol 1993;161:147–52.

[6] Wiersma F, Sramek A, Holscher HC. US features of the normal appendix and surrounding area in children. Radiology 2005;235:1018–22.

[7] Quillin SP, Siegel MJ. Appendicitis: efficacy of color Doppler sonography. Radiology 1994;191:557–60.

[8] Quillin SP, Siegel MJ, Coffin CM. Acute appendicitis in children: value of sonography in detecting perforation. Am J Roentgenol 1992;159:1265–8.

[9] Borushok KF, Jeffrey RB Jr, Laing FC, et al. Sonographic diagnosis of perforation in patients with acute appendicitis. Am J Roentgenol 1990;154:275–8.

[10] Hayden CK Jr, Kuchelmeister J, Lipscomb TS. Sonography of acute appendicitis in childhood: perforation versus nonperforation. J Ultrasound Med 1992;11:209–16.

[11] Hahn HB, Hoepner FU, Kalle T, et al. Sonography of acute appendicitis in children: 7 years experience. Pediatr Radiol 1998;28:147–51.

[12] Dilley A, Wesson D, Munden M, et al. The impact of ultrasound examinations on the management of children with suspected appendicitis: a 3-year analysis. J Pediatr Surg 2001;36:303–8.

[13] Sivit CJ. Controversies in emergency radiology: acute appendicitis in children—the case for CT. Emerg Radiol 2004;10:238–40.

[14] Applegate KE, Sivit CJ, Salvator AE, et al. Effect of cross-sectional imaging on negative appendectomy and perforation rates in children. Radiology 2001;220:103–7.

[15] Kaiser S, Frenckner B, Jorulf HK. Suspected appendicitis in children: US and CT—a prospective randomized study. Radiology 2002;223:633–8.

[16] Sivit CJ, Applegate KE, Stallion A, et al. Imaging evaluation of suspected appendicitis in a pediatric population: effectiveness of sonography versus CT. Am J Roentgenol 2000;175:977–80.

[17] Garcia Pena BM, Taylor GA, Fishman SJ, et al. Effect of an imaging protocol on clinical outcomes among pediatric patients with appendicitis. Pediatrics 2002;110:1088–93.

[18] Puig S, Hörmann M, Rebhandl W, et al. US as a primary diagnostic tool in relation to negative appendectomy: six years experience. Radiology 2003;226:101–4.

[19] Garcia Pena BM, Taylor GA, Fishman SJ, et al. Costs and effectiveness of ultrasonography and limited computed tomography for diagnosing appendicitis in children. Pediatrics 2000;106:672–6.

[20] Garcia Pena BM, Mandl KD, Kraus SJ, et al. Ultrasonography and limited computed tomography in the diagnosis and management of appendicitis in children. JAMA 1999;282:1041–6.

[21] Vayner N, Coret A, Polliack G, et al. Mesenteric lymphadenopathy in children examined by US for chronic and/or recurrent abdominal pain. Pediatr Radiol 2003;33:864–7.

[22] Karmazyn B, Werner EA, Rejaie B, et al. Mesenteric lymph nodes in children: what is normal? Pediatr Radiol 2005;35:774–7.

[23] Puylaert JB. Mesenteric adenitis and acute terminal ileitis: US evaluation using graded compression. Radiology 1986;161:691–5.

[24] Eshed I, Gorenstein A, Serour F, et al. Intussusception in children: can we rely on screening sonography performed by junior residents? Pediatr Radiol 2004;34:134–7.

[25] Henrikson S, Blane CE, Koujok K, et al. The effect of screening sonography on the positive rate of enemas for intussusception. Pediatr Radiol 2003;33:190–3.

[26] Daneman A, Navarro O. Intussusception. Part 1: a review of diagnostic approaches. Pediatr Radiol 2003;33:79–85.

[27] Shanbhogue RL, Hussain SM, Meradji M, et al. Ultrasonography is accurate enough for the diagnosis of intussusception. J Pediatr Surg 1994;29:324–7. [discussion 327–8].

[28] Verschelden P, Filiatrault D, Garel L, et al. Intussusception in children: reliability of US in diagnosis—a prospective study. Radiology 1992;184:741–4.

[29] del-Pozo G, Albillos JC, Tejedor D. Intussusception: US findings with pathologic correlation—the crescent-in-doughnut sign. Radiology 1996;199:688–92.

[30] Koumanidou C, Vakaki M, Pitsoulakis G, et al. Sonographic detection of lymph nodes in the intussusception of infants and young children: clinical evaluation and hydrostatic reduction. Am J Roentgenol 2002;178:445–50.

[31] del-Pozo G, Gonzalez-Spinola J, Gomez-Anson B, et al. Intussusception: trapped peritoneal fluid detected with US—relationship to reducibility and ischemia. Radiology 1996;201:379–83.

[32] Lim HK, Bae SH, Lee KH, et al. Assessment of reducibility of ileocolic intussusception in children: usefulness of color Doppler sonography. Radiology 1994;191:781–5.

[33] Kim JH. US features of transient small bowel intussusception in pediatric patients. Korean J Radiol 2004;5:178–84.

[34] Navarro O, Daneman A. Intussusception. Part 3: diagnosis and management of those with an identifiable or predisposing cause and those that reduce spontaneously. Pediatr Radiol 2004;34:305–12. quiz 369.

[35] Woo SK, Kim JS, Suh SJ, et al. Childhood intussusception: US-guided hydrostatic reduction. Radiology 1992;182:77–80.

[36] Yoon CH, Kim HJ, Goo HW. Intussusception in children: US-guided pneumatic reduction—initial experience. Radiology 2001;218:85–8.

[37] Teele RL, Henschke CI, Tapper D. The radiographic and ultrasonographic evaluation of enteric duplication cysts. Pediatr Radiol 1980;10:9–14.

[38] Macpherson RI. Gastrointestinal tract duplications: clinical, pathologic, etiologic, and radiologic considerations. Radiographics 1993;13:1063–80.

[39] Cheng G, Soboleski D, Daneman A, et al. Sonographic pitfalls in the diagnosis of enteric duplication cysts. Am J Roentgenol 2005;184:521–5.

[40] Bower RJ, Sieber WK, Kiesewetter WB. Alimentary tract duplications in children. Ann Surg 1978;188:669–74.

[41] Faure C, Belarbi N, Mougenot JF, et al. Ultrasonographic assessment of inflammatory bowel disease in children: comparison with ileocolonoscopy. J Pediatr 1997;130:147–51.

[42] Haber HP, Busch A, Ziebach R, et al. Bowel wall thickness measured by ultrasound as a marker of Crohn's disease activity in children. Lancet 2000; 355:1239–40.

[43] Chang WL, Yang YH, Lin YT, et al. Gastrointestinal manifestations in Henoch-Schönlein purpura: a review of 261 patients. Acta Paediatr 2004;93:1427–31.

[44] Bomelburg T, Claasen U, von Lengerke HJ. Intestinal ultrasonographic findings in Schönlein-Henoch syndrome. Eur J Pediatr 1991;150:158–60.

[45] Ozdemir H, Isik S, Buyan N, et al. Sonographic demonstration of intestinal involvement in Henoch-Schönlein syndrome. Eur J Radiol 1995; 20:32–4.

[46] Levy AD, Hobbs CM. From the archives of the AFIP. Meckel diverticulum: radiologic features with pathologic correlation. Radiographics 2004;24:565–87.

[47] Baldisserotto M, Maffazzoni DR, Dora MD. Sonographic findings of Meckel's diverticulitis in children. Am J Roentgenol 2003;180:425–8.

[48] Traubici J, Daneman A, Wales P, et al. Mesenteric lymphatic malformation associated with small-bowel volvulus—two cases and a review of the literature. Pediatr Radiol 2002;32:362–5.

[49] Baldisserotto M, Maffazzoni DR, Dora MD. Omental infarction in children: color Doppler sonography correlated with surgery and pathology findings. Am J Roentgenol 2005;184:156–62.

[50] Grattan-Smith JD, Blews DE, Brand T. Omental infarction in pediatric patients: sonographic and CT findings. Am J Roentgenol 2002;178:1537–9.

[51] Nimkin K, Lebowitz RL, Share JC, et al. Urolithiasis in a children's hospital: 1985–1990. Urol Radiol 1992;14:139–43.

[52] Strouse PJ, Bates DG, Bloom DA, et al. Noncontrast thin-section helical CT of urinary tract calculi in children. Pediatr Radiol 2002;32: 326–32.

[53] Smith SL, Somers JM, Broderick N, et al. The role of the plain radiograph and renal tract ultrasound in the management of children with renal tract calculi. Clin Radiol 2000;55:708–10.

[54] Yu JS, Kim KW, Lee HJ, et al. Urachal remnant diseases: spectrum of CT and US findings. Radiographics 2001;21:451–61.

[55] Blask AR, Sanders RC, Rock JA. Obstructed uterovaginal anomalies: demonstration with sonography. Part II. Teenagers. Radiology 1991;179: 84–8.

[56] Baltarowich OH, Kurtz AB, Pasto ME, et al. The spectrum of sonographic findings in hemorrhagic ovarian cysts. Am J Roentgenol 1987; 148:901–5.

[57] de Silva KS, Kanumakala S, Grover SR, et al. Ovarian lesions in children and adolescents— an 11-year review. J Pediatr Endocrinol Metab 2004;17:951–7.

[58] Surratt JT, Siegel MJ. Imaging of pediatric ovarian masses. Radiographics 1991;11:533–48.

[59] Ammerman S, Shafer MA, Snyder D. Ectopic pregnancy in adolescents: a clinical review for pediatricians. J Pediatr 1990;117:677–86.

[60] Dialani V, Levine D. Ectopic pregnancy: a review. Ultrasound Q 2004;20:105–17.

[61] Frates MC, Laing FC. Sonographic evaluation of ectopic pregnancy: an update. Am J Roentgenol 1995;165:251–9.

[62] Bellah RD, Rosenberg HK. Transvaginal ultrasound in a children's hospital: is it worthwhile? Pediatr Radiol 1991;21:570–4.

[63] Banikarim C, Chacko MR. Pelvic inflammatory disease in adolescents. Adolesc Med Clin 2004; 15:273–85. [viii.].

[64] Bulas DI, Ahlstrom PA, Sivit CJ, et al. Pelvic inflammatory disease in the adolescent: comparison of transabdominal and transvaginal sonographic evaluation. Radiology 1992;183: 435–9.

[65] Godfrey H, Abernethy L, Boothroyd A. Torsion of an ovarian cyst mimicking enteric duplication cyst on transabdominal ultrasound: two cases. Pediatr Radiol 1998;28:171–3.

[66] Graif M, Itzchak Y. Sonographic evaluation of ovarian torsion in childhood and adolescence. Am J Roentgenol 1988;150:647–9.

[67] Stark JE, Siegel MJ. Ovarian torsion in prepubertal and pubertal girls: sonographic findings. Am J Roentgenol 1994;163:1479–82.

RADIOLOGIC
CLINICS
OF NORTH AMERICA

Radiol Clin N Am 44 (2006) 925–935

ELSEVIER
SAUNDERS

Intraoperative Laparoscopic Ultrasound

Suvranu Ganguli, MD[a,b,*], Jonathan B. Kruskal, MD, PhD[a,b],
Darren D. Brennan, MD[a,b], Robert A. Kane, MD, FACR[a,b]

As minimally invasive surgery and laparoscopic alternatives to open surgical procedures continue to increase, the demand for and use of intraoperative laparoscopic ultrasound (LUS) techniques also are increasing steadily. The benefit of scanning directly on the surface of intra-abdominal organs, structures, and pathology and the improved spatial and contrast resolution seen in open intraoperative ultrasound (IOUS) [1] can be transferred to laparoscopic procedures. LUS shows beneficial applications in evaluating normal structures and pathology within the liver, pancreas, biliary tract, and gallbladder [2–4]. There also are reports of LUS improving localization and laparoscopic staging of intra-abdominal tumors [5–8]. The need for specially designed equipment, especially special transducers for LUS, traditionally has been the greatest obstacle to its widespread use. With the increasing demand and use of laparoscopy and LUS, however, there continues to be improving technology and exciting new possibilities.

Laparoscopic probe design

The overriding stipulation for laparoscopic probes is that the diameter of the imaging crystal and shaft must to be small enough to be inserted through a standard laparoscopic port 10 to 11 mm in diameter. Transducer technology has progressed substantially from the first reports of LUS, where investigators used A-mode transducers to visualize intra-abdominal organs and assist in the diagnosis of intra-abdominal pathology [9,10]. The limited amount of information obtained with the primitive A-mode technology resulted in limited applicability of this technique. The subsequent development of real-time B-mode ultrasound and improved

This article was originally published in *Ultrasound Clinics* 1:3, July 2006.
[a] Department of Radiology, Beth Israel Deaconess Medical Center, 330 Brookline Avenue, Boston, MA 02215, USA
[b] Harvard Medical School, Boston, MA, USA
* Corresponding author. Department of Radiology, Beth Israel Deaconess Medical Center, 330 Brookline Avenue, Boston, MA 02215.
E-mail address: sganguli@caregroup.harvard.edu (S. Ganguli).

doi:10.1016/j.rcl.2006.10.020

miniaturization technology made the laparoscopic approach more feasible. Early probes also used a rotating radial probe [11], but the subsequent development of linear array and curved array, high-frequency probes has resulted in superior image resolution.

The miniaturization of the crystal size previously has led to probes with extremely small field of views. The small field of view of laparoscopic probes compared with standard ultrasound probes remains an obstacle, but the development and improvement of linear array and curved array probes have improved this constraint significantly. Optimal image crystal lengths for intra-abdominal laparoscopic probes range from 1.5 to 4 cm. Longer crystal lengths help provide larger images that can shorten scanning time of larger organs, such as the liver. The curved array probes also provide a more familiar sector-style image, allowing for easier orientation and greater visualization of deep anatomy in any one field.

In the authors' experience, probe frequencies centered at 5 MHz permit adequate depth of penetration to image the entire liver. Probes now are designed with multifrequency options or broadband technology, which allows a range of frequencies. This allows more flexibility in penetration to suit the specific intraoperative imaging needs. Higher frequencies of 7 to 10 MHz are more suitable for imaging the gallbladder, common bile duct (CBD),

and pancreas. These improvements in probe technology, coupled with the expansion in computer power, have enabled the design and development of laparoscopic probes that now have the same image quality, resolution, Doppler, and color flow imaging capacities as standard ultrasound probes.

In addition to the miniaturization required of laparoscopic probes, a radically different probe design is needed to optimize use in a laparoscopic setting. Laparoscopic probes must be mounted at the end of a long shaft, measuring 20 to 30 cm in length, to facilitate imaging organs, structure, and pathology some distance away from the entry site on the abdominal wall (Fig. 1). Early probes were mounted on the end of rigid shafts designed to be passed through standard laparoscopic ports. Recent probes are designed to be more flexible and maneuverable at the transducer tip. At minimum, flexion and extension of the imaging crystal now are available and newer systems provide rightward and leftward steering. The flexible imaging portion of the probe allows for good tissue contact necessary for acoustic coupling to be maintained in a gas-filled peritoneal cavity. Maintaining surface contact with curved or irregularly shaped organs and mastering a maneuverable laparoscopic probe require practice and experience. Without optimal probe flexibility, adequate imaging may require filling the abdominal cavity with sterile water or saline and imaging through the fluid.

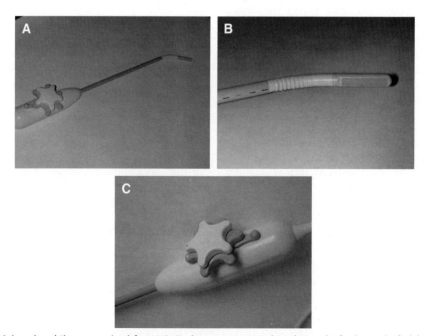

Fig. 1. Special probes (*A*) are required for LUS. Probes are mounted at the end of a long shaft (*B*) to facilitate imaging organs, structure, and pathology some distance away from the entry site on the abdominal wall. Flexion and extension of the probe is performed by turning dials (*C*) on the proximal shaft outside the patient.

Transducer sterilization

Sterile sheaths similar to those used on standard ultrasound probes for IOUS can be used during LUS. Because of the nature of laparoscopic procedures, however, with repetitive insertion and removal of probes through ports and using inserted tools, such as the laparoscopic instruments, for manipulation of intra-abdominal organs and structures, sheaths continually run a high risk of tearing during use. For these reasons, sterilization capability is a more optimal requirement for laparoscopic probes compared with standard ultrasound probes.

Specially designed strong sterile sheaths are used for LUS and should have a snug fit to the transducer, if used, to avoid being torn during insertion. These sheaths are long, typically approximately 1.5 m, so that the entire length of the cord can be covered. Sterile saline or gel must be used between the tip and the sheath to avoid artifact from trapped air. If sterile sheaths are used, it is still advisable to soak the probe for some time in a sterilizing solution, as the potential for tearing of the sheath and contamination of the surgical field remains.

Newer-generation laparoscopic probes are designed to be compatible with modern sterilization methods. Ideally, the entire ultrasound probe except the electronic connector is sterilized. Low-temperature hydrogen peroxide gas plasma sterilization techniques (Sterrad, Advanced Sterilization Products, Irvine, California) can complete an entire sterilization cycle in 1 to 2 hours. These sterilization techniques are safe to use with heat-sensitive equipment and can help avoid use of sterile sheaths.

Intraoperative scanning techniques

Selection of port placement is highly dependent on the target organ or area requiring LUS evaluation (Fig. 2). Often surgeons need to create port sites for the laparoscope and the laparoscopic instruments before using LUS. Optimal placement of a port transducer site, however, usually is several centimeters away from the area to allow room to maneuver the probe freely. Frequently, the LUS probe and the laparoscope (usually in a periumbilical port) must be reversed or multiple ports must be created to reach all areas necessary with the LUS probe. If the laparoscopic procedure has the potential of being converted to an open procedure, it is optimal to include port sites within the line of a subsequent incision.

Ensuring that the ports are airtight before inserting the LUS probe is important to maintain the iatrogenic pneumoperitoneum of laparoscopy (Fig. 3). If a standard 10-mm LUS probe is inserted, make sure that the 10- to 11-mm adjustable port is

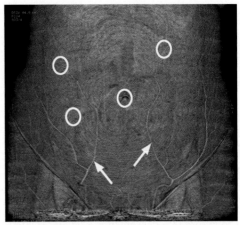

Fig. 2. Localizing the site for port insertion requires avoiding important subcutaneous vessels (*arrows*). Common insertion sites (shown as rings) are in the left and right subcostal, right lower quadrant and umbilical regions.

set to the appropriate 10-mm size to prevent leakage of gas. After port insertion, it is important again to assess for leakage of gas around the port and address problems as they arise. The sterile transducer must be inserted carefully though the port with direct laparoscopic visualization to ensure safe delivery to the region of interest (Fig. 4). As there is no tactile sensation available to the LUS operator, direct laparoscopic visualization of the probe is imperative at all times during scanning to avoid solid organ or vessel injury. It is necessary always to be cognizant of the location of the transducer tip on the laparoscopic camera images—looking at the ultrasound image alone may cause inadvertent injury (Fig. 5).

Even though the peritoneal cavity is distended with gas, natural organ surface moisture usually is sufficient to permit adequate acoustic coupling and optimal image quality. If necessary, sterile saline can be introduced onto the organ surface to

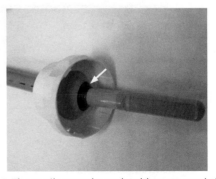

Fig. 3. The sterile transducer should create an airtight seal as it passes through the port. Note the circular valve (*arrow*), which ensures that the port is airtight.

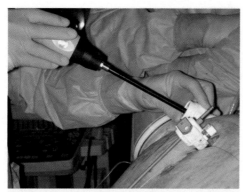

Fig. 4. The sterile transducer must be inserted carefully through the port, keeping an eye on the monitor to ensure safe delivery into a region of interest. If a sheath is used, very gentle insertion is essential to avoid tearing.

enhance acoustic coupling. As discussed previously, if an overlying sheath is used, sterile saline or gel must be used between the tip and the sheath to avoid artifact from trapped air.

The optimal choice of imaging frequency is dependent on the target organ or organ system. The gallbladder, extrahepatic CBD, and pancreas can be imaged successfully at a 7-MHz frequency. The liver, however, is imaged optimally at a 5-MHz frequency, which penetrates to a depth of 10 to 12 cm rather than a depth of approximately 6 cm at 7 MHz. Using the lower, 5-MHz frequency does not impair the ability of visualize small lesions but does facilitate complete scanning of the liver from the anterior surface of the liver [2]. This way, using the undersurface of the liver for scanning can be avoided. The undersurface of the liver is much more irregular and less accessible, causing imaging from this side to be more challenging technically.

Compared with IOUS, LUS takes substantially more time to image the same structures because of the small crystal size and field of view. The curved

array sector scanners give an impression of a large field of view, but this is true only at depths of several centimeters. The near field is limited by the transducer length, which may be as short as 1.5 to 2 cm. Therefore, complete evaluation of the liver requires overlapping these 2-cm near-field images across the entire length and breath of liver, which can be a time-consuming process [2].

Moreover, scanning becomes more difficult as the probe must be manipulated along a pivot point where the proximal shaft is fixed at the insertion port. The probe can be moved vertically in a cephalocaudal direction, but when it is moved laterally or medially, the shaft begins to pivot and the plane of view changes from a sagittal plane to an evermore oblique plane. With extreme pivoting, the plane of view may be closer to transverse than sagittal. This constantly changing plane of view can be disorienting, particularly to inexperienced observers. Constant reference to the orientation of the probe on the laparoscopic image can be helpful in attempting to overlap the imaging fields and obtain complete evaluation of the liver [2].

Before actually scanning, it is imperative to discuss with the clinicians and establish the information required by LUS. As patients are under general anesthesia and because of the high costs involved in an operating room setting, it is best to limit the amount of time used for LUS scanning to obtain the information required. It also is extremely beneficial to review any preoperative imaging, including previous ultrasound, CT, or MR imaging, before entering the operating room. Having these images directly available for consultation while in the operating room can help reduce overall study time and help focus the examination.

Operating room ergonomics

Optimal positioning of the monitors in relation to the probes can minimize difficulties and enhance

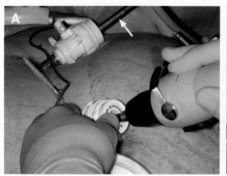
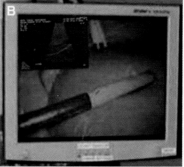

Fig. 5. Once inserted into the peritoneal cavity (*A*), the ultrasound probe (in the near field) must be watched continuously via the laparoscopic camera probe (*arrow*). Direct laparoscopic visualization of the ultrasound probe on the monitor (*B*) is essential at all times to avoid solid organ or vessel injury.

the experience for LUS operators significantly. The monitors should be placed in a location that is natural for operators to manipulate the transducer while simultaneously viewing the monitors. Placing monitors in positions that force operators to contort their bodies uncomfortably while manipulating the transducer should be avoided. The display monitors should be large enough and placed close enough to operators so that subtle abnormalities during scanning can be visualized easily.

Moreover, because operators view two screens simultaneously, a split screen (picture-in-picture) presentation using an electronic beam-splitting device is the optimal operating room scenario. These split-screen setups usually can adjust which real-time feed, the laparoscopic or ultrasound images, is displayed as the larger image and can be exchanged as needed. Displaying the laparoscopic and ultrasound images on the same monitor facilitates scanning and interpretation and at the same time reduces the risk of solid organ or vascular injury by the transducer.

Clinical applications of laparoscopic ultrasound

Laparoscopic ultrasound of the liver

As discussed previously, the liver is imaged best at a center frequency of 5 MHz, allowing for depth of penetration of 10 to 12 cm. Unlike standard IOUS, LUS takes considerably more time to scan the entire liver, as the near field is limited strictly by the length of the crystal. Complete scanning takes approximately 15 minutes with LUS versus 5 minutes with IOUS. Each survey of the liver should be done in an organized and systematic fashion, with the intention of overlapping each sequential imaging field completely so that the entire liver parenchyma is assessed (Fig. 6).

In a typical survey of the liver, a right subcostal port placement is used with direct and continuous visualization with the laparoscope from the standard periumbilical port. The LUS probe is passed as far cephalad as possible while the operator scans across the dome of the right lobe of the liver from

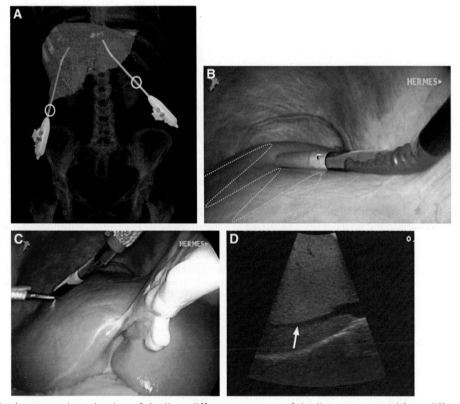

Fig. 6. For laparoscopic evaluation of the liver, different segments of the liver are accessed from different ports (*A*). Imaging is performed (*B*) with overlapping transverse scans (dotted lines). When imaging the hepatic dome (*C*), the probe must be positioned to the right of the fat-containing falciform ligament and flexed over the dome. In this way, structures, such as an accessory superior right hepatic vein (*D*) in segment VII (*arrow*), can be imaged.

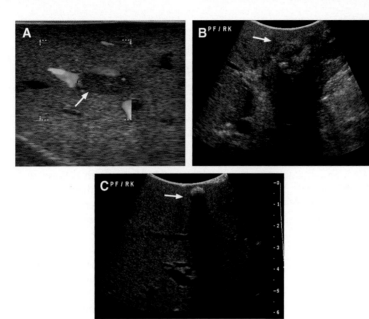

Fig. 7. LUS can be an effective tool for intraoperative oncologic staging. During a laparoscopic bowel resection for colon cancer (*A*), LUS identified an unexpected solitary hypoechoic lesion (*arrow*) in segment VII of the liver. LUS-guided biopsy confirmed metastatic tumor. LUS in a different patient who had mucinous colorectal metastases (*B*) demonstrated an ill-defined calcified mass arising in segment III of the liver (*arrows*). LUS at the time (*C*) also identified a calcified biopsy-proved metastatic subcapsular lesion (*arrow*) in segment V.

left to right. The falciform ligament and ligamentum teres are barriers when imaging the left liver lobe via a right subcostal port and limit the medial extent of the sweep. Systematic scanning of the right and medial left lobes then are performed by withdrawing the probe approximately 2 cm in between overlapping sweeps across the liver.

Imaging of the left lateral segment requires either incision of the falciform ligament or switching ports between the laparoscopic and LUS probes or forming a separate LUS probe insertion via a left subcostal port. Usually the periumbilical port is sufficient to access segments 1 to 3. Once the probe is in position at the dome of the left lateral segment, systematic scanning is performed again from left to right, with the falciform ligament again creating the barrier for the medial extent of the sweep.

The most common hepatic application of LUS is tumor staging. Laparoscopy often is used for preoperative staging of primary hepatic and metastatic tumors to optimally select candidates for resection (Fig. 7). Laparoscopy has proved superior to conventional preoperative imaging in staging of hepatocellular carcinoma, with more recent reports that laparoscopy with LUS provides superior information for the diagnosis and pretreatment staging of primary and metastatic hepatic tumors [6,12,13].

Obviously, deep liver tumor nodules cannot be detected with the laparoscope itself. LUS can reveal additional hepatic masses, metastatic lymphadenopathy, and vascular invasion not visualized on standard preoperative staging. Additional lesions disclosed on LUS generally are small, frequently less than 1 cm in diameter and, therefore, below the limit of resolution of most preoperative

imaging modalities. Such findings can influence surgical decision-making and some studies have gone as far as to recommend routine use of LUS of the liver during all laparoscopic oncologic surgeries [13,14].

Other uses for LUS in the liver include accurate localization of tumors to specific lobes or segments and assessment of contiguous vascular and biliary structures. Invasions of bile ducts and the portal and hepatic venous system are well demonstrated. Accessory vascular supply and venous drainage to and from the liver can influence the type and extent of resection to be performed greatly. LUS may be required to characterize vascular anastomoses after liver transplantation, to confirm patency of intrahepatic vessels, and to guide cautery on the liver capsule when these surface markers are used to guide deeper incisions. Replaced or accessory right and left hepatic arteries and accessory hepatic veins can be well demonstrated. LUS also can characterize lesions that are inconclusive on other imaging modalities, potentially influencing patient treatment. The ability to further characterize lesions using LUS may be most beneficial in determining benign abnormalities, such as focal fatty infiltration, focal areas of fatty sparing in a diffusely fatty liver, hemangiomas, or cysts from metastatic lesions.

Laparoscopic ultrasound of the gallbladder and bile ducts

The gallbladder and extrahepatic bile ducts usually can be imaged satisfactorily from a right subcostal port or from the periumbilical port. Also, from the left subcostal port, a so-called "Mickey Mouse"

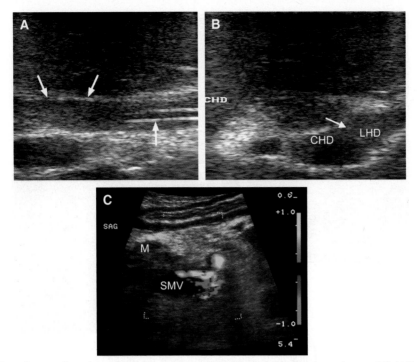

Fig. 8. In this patient undergoing planned resection of extrahepatic cholangiocarcinoma (*A*), LUS documented extent of involvement of the CBD (*angled arrows*). Tumor surrounds a previously placed biliary stent (*small vertical arrow*). Tumor extension (*B*) beyond the common hepatic duct (CHD) up into the left hepatic duct (LHD) (*arrow*) also was identified. In a different patient who had cholangiocarcinoma (*C*), LUS was used to localize the mass (M) and, using color flow, to confirm invasion of the superior mesenteric vein (SMV).

appearance of the ducts and adjacent hepatic artery is noted. The gallbladder is imaged best through the liver using a 5- or 7-MHz transducer. The extrahepatic bile ducts often are imaged best at 7 MHz though a compressed duodenum or gastric antrum, because near-field reverberation artifact limits sensitivity when the transducer is placed directly on the ducts. The distal-most portion of the CBD is visualized by imaging the head of the pancreas. Color flow images are helpful for distinguishing the CBD from the portal vein and should be used routinely. Although the cystic duct usually is not well visualized on preoperative imaging, it can be identified routinely on LUS, including where it joins the CBD. This visualization can be helpful in identifying aberrant anatomy, such as a low insertion of the cystic duct into the CBD, which otherwise is unnoticed.

As laparoscopic cholecystectomy has become the standard of care in gallbladder disease, the use of LUS during these procedures is an increasing possibility. LUS can be a viable alternative to laparoscopic cholangiography. Common duct stones and strictures are visualized easily on LUS and it is recommended as the primary screening procedure for bile duct calculi because of its safety, speed, and cost-effectiveness [15]. Consequently, the routine use of laparoscopic cholangiography is not advised, because the yield of positive studies has proved low [16]. In the authors' experience, however, although LUS is available and efficacious, patients who have suspicious clinical, laboratory, or imaging findings for CBD abnormalities usually are referred for preoperative endoscopic retrograde cholangiopancreatography instead. As technology and experience with LUS advances, this could be an area for increased use in the future.

Further applications of LUS include oncologic staging of gallbladder and bile duct tumors, such as gallbladder carcinoma and cholangiocarcinoma (Fig. 8). The extent of invasion into the adjacent liver bed is difficult for surgeons to detect by inspection and palpation and can be portrayed well by IOUS [17]. Apart from identifying subtle liver metastasis (described previously), LUS can help define local extent of tumor and the involvement or sparing of ductal systems. LUS can help distinguish biliary sludge from intraluminal tumor with the use of targeted Doppler and color flow imaging. Moreover, benign strictures and malignant obstructions of the biliary tract can be defined further to help plan the type of biliary bypass procedure to be performed.

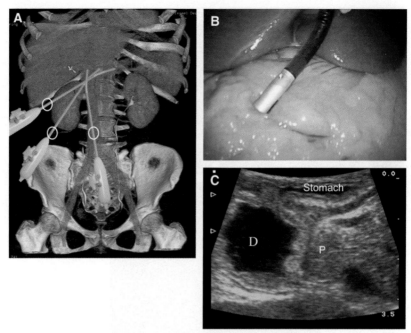

Fig. 9. For imaging the bile ducts and pancreatic head, probes (*A*) can be inserted in through right upper quadrant, right lower quadrant, or umbilical ports. The pancreatic body (*B*) can be imaged via a right subcostal port, typically imaged through the compressed stomach. When imaging the head (*C*) of the pancreas (P), the second part of the duodenum (D) is seen lateral to the head.

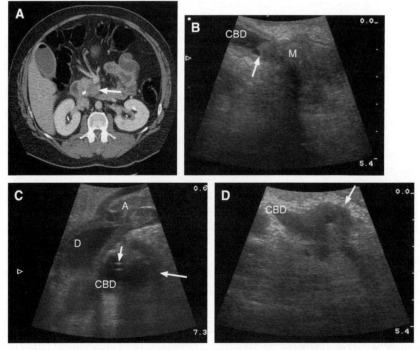

Fig. 10. Contrast-enhanced axial CT image (*A*) demonstrates a pancreatic head mass (*arrow*) encircling the CBD. At surgery, LUS (*B*) was used to localize the mass (M) and to document direct extension into the CBD (*arrow*). In a different patient (*C*), imaging through the compressed gastric antrum (A), an adenocarcinoma of the ampulla (*large arrow*) was identified in the head of the pancreas. Note the adjacent duodenum (D) and dilated CBD with a biliary stent (*small arrow*). LUS also showed (*D*) extension of the tumor (*arrow*), surrounding and extending into the CBD.

Laparoscopic ultrasound of the pancreas

The pancreas, from the head and uncinate process to the tail, can be imaged successfully at a 7-MHz frequency. The LUS approach to the pancreas is best through a right upper or left upper quadrant port, allowing the probe to be oriented along the long axis of the pancreas in a relatively transverse plane (Fig. 9). This allows for better orientation than attempting to image in the sagittal oblique plane across the short axis of the pancreas. The periumbilical port also can be useful in imaging the head/neck and uncinate process using a sagittal approach. Scanning can be performed directly on the pancreatic surface or through the overlying omentum. Occasionally, the lateral segment of the liver can provide an acoustic window to the pancreatic body and tail.

The main application for LUS in regard to pancreatic surgery is in conjunction with laparoscopic staging of pancreatic and periampullary tumors (Fig. 10). Although preoperative ultrasound, CT, and MR imaging can demonstrate vascular invasion or hepatic metastatic disease successfully, a significant number of patients who have advanced disease remain incompletely staged before surgery. Studies show the improved staging of pancreatic and perimpullary tumors by laparoscopy with LUS versus standard preoperative imaging methods [7,18].

LUS of the pancreas also is described as a sensitive and successful method in localizing islet cell tumors (Fig. 11) [19,20]. This method may be important particularly for small lesions localized to the body or tail of the pancreas, because laparoscopic partial pancreatic resections can be performed. Laparoscopy with LUS is reported to contribute significantly to the differential diagnosis of pancreatic cystic neoplasms [21,22], helping delineate serous microcystic adenomas, mucinous cystadenomas, or cystadenocarcinomas and intraductal papillary mucinous neoplasms of the pancreas (Fig. 12). LUS imaging also can help identify the extent of pseudocysts and pancreatic ductal abnormalities in patients who have pancreatitis. Transgastric LUS imaging can be used to facilitate laparoscopic cystgastrostomy.

Other applications

As more and more surgical procedures move to laparoscopic approaches, the possible applications for LUS continue to increase. There are reports of improved localization of intra-abdominal tumors using LUS during planned laparoscopic resections.

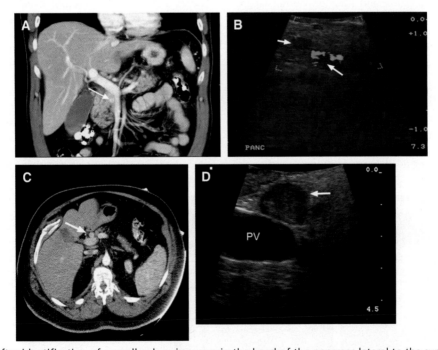

Fig. 11. After identification of a small enhancing mass in the head of the pancreas lateral to the superior mesenteric vein (*arrow*) on a contrast-enhanced CT scan (*A*), LUS (*B*) was performed to confirm and characterize the mass (*small arrow*) and depict proximity of the mass to the adjacent superior mesenteric vein (*large arrow*). Based on the LUS findings, laparoscopy was converted to an open procedure and resection revealed an islet cell tumor. In another patient, a 3-mm enhancing lesion (*C*) was identified on a contrast-enhanced CT scan (*arrow*). LUS (*D*) was used to localize the lesion (*arrow*) to show absence of portal vein (PV) invasion and to guide surgical resection, which showed a nonfunctioning insulinoma.

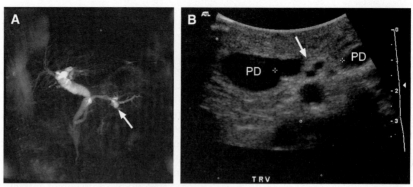

Fig. 12. After identification of a cystic mass (*A*) in the body of the pancreas on this coronal T2-weighted magnetic resonance cholangiopancreatography image (*arrow*), LUS (*B*) was used to localize the mass (*arrow*) and guide the resection. Note the dilated pancreatic ducts (PD) proximal and distal to the mass. Pathology confirmed that this was an intraductal papillary mucinous neoplasm.

For example, LUS shows improved localization of adrenal tumors by defining the relationship to adjacent structures and providing confirmation that larger tumors are amenable to laparoscopic resection [23]. Reports of LUS use in gynecologic surgery also are increasing, with studies describing improved laparoscopic ovarian tumor localization and staging [24] and management of ovarian cysts and adnexal masses [25]. LUS also is used to evaluate ureteral location and function during laparoscopic gynecologic surgery to help lower the incidence of intraoperative ureteral complications [26]. The full and complete use of LUS remains to be seen.

Biopsy and percutaneous ablation guidance

Superficial and larger deep tumors within organs can be biopsied readily under direct laparoscopic visualization or with LUS assistance (Fig. 13). Traditional LUS-guided biopsies require placing the transducer over the site to be biopsied followed by percutaneous insertion of a long needle through the abdominal wall down to the level of the transducer. This technique can make small, deep lesions difficult to biopsy because of the considerable distances between the needle insertion in the anterior abdominal wall and the location of the LUS probe. When lesions are located in deep positions, it may be necessary to vent some gas from the peritoneal cavity once the transducer is placed on the biopsy site to minimize the distance. Newer-generation laparoscopic probes, however, are designed with puncture and biopsy guides, making small, deep lesions easier to biopsy under LUS guidance.

LUS also has the potential to guide minimally invasive tumor ablations, although experience thus far is limited. Minimally invasive oncology therapies technology, such as radiofrequency ablation, microwave ablation, and cryosurgery, continue to be developed and used. With the improved tumor localization provided by LUS, evolution to LUS-guided minimally invasive therapies is a logical next step.

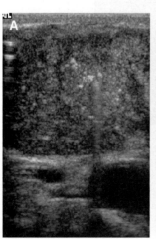

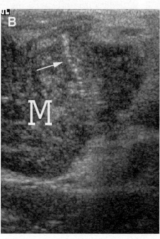

Fig. 13. (*A,B*) A percutaneous needle (*arrow*) is inserted into a hypoechoic pancreatic mass (M) adjacent to the transducer for LUS-guided pancreas biopsy. Although adenocarcinoma was suspected from preoperative imaging studies, pathology revealed lymphocytic sclerosing pancreatitis.

Summary

As more open surgical procedures move to laparoscopic approaches, the demand for LUS continues to increase. New improvements in technology and equipment already have advanced LUS from its experimental beginnings to the point of routine clinical applications. Applications in the liver, pancreas, gallbladder, and biliary tree are described, with further applications in gynecologic surgery also reported. The applications in LUS-guided biopsies and minimally invasive therapies remain to be perfected. An operator learning curve remains, however, and mastery of LUS requires familiarity with the special equipment and scanning techniques. But as technology and the widespread use continue to advance, the full range and importance of LUS applications no doubt will increase.

References

[1] Kane RA, Hughs LA, Cua EJ, et al. The impact of intraoperative ultrasonography on surgery for liver neoplasms. J Ultrasound Med 1994;13:1–6.

[2] Kane RA. Laparoscopic ultrasound. In: Kane RA, editor. Intraoperative, laparoscopic, and endoluminal ultrasound. Philadelphia: Churchill Livingstone; 1999. p. 90–105.

[3] Ascher SM, Evans SRT, Goldberg JA, et al. Intraoperative bile duct sonography during laparoscopic cholecystectomy: experience with a 12.5 MHz catheter based US probe. Radiology 1992; 185:493–6.

[4] Yamamoto M, Stiegmann GV, Durham J, et al. Laparoscopy-guided intracorporeal ultrasound accurately delineates hepatobiliary anatomy. Surg Endosc 1993;7:325–30.

[5] Goletti O, Celona G, Galatioto C, et al. Is laparoscopic sonography a reliable and sensitive procedure for staging colorectal cancer? A comparative study. Surg Endosc 1998;12:1236–41.

[6] Montorsi M, Santambrogio R, Bianchi P, et al. Laparoscopy with laparoscopic ultrasound for pretreatment staging of hepatocellular carcinoma: a prospective study. J Gastrointest Surg 2001;5: 312–5.

[7] Doran HE, Bosonnet L, Connor S, et al. Laparoscopy and laparoscopic ultrasound in the evaluation of pancreatic and periampullary tumours. Dig Surg 2004;21:305–13.

[8] Vollmer CM, Drebin JA, Middleton WD, et al. Utility of staging laparoscopy in subsets of peripancreatic and biliary malignancies. Ann Surg 2002;235:1–7.

[9] Yamakawa K, Naito S, Azuma K, et al. Laparoscopic diagnosis of the intra-abdominal organs. Jpn J Gastroenterol 1958;55:741–7.

[10] Yamakawa K, Yoshioka A, Shimizu K, et al. Laparoechography: an ultrasonic diagnosis under laparoscopic observation. Jpn Med Ultrasonics 1964;2:26.

[11] Fornari F, Civardi G, Cavanna L, et al. Laparoscopic ultrasonography in the study of liver diseases. Preliminary results. Surg Endosc 1989;3:33–7.

[12] Foroutani A, Garland AM, Berber E, et al. Laparoscopic ultrasound vs triphasic computed tomography for detecting liver tumors. Arch Surg 2000; 135:933–8.

[13] Thaler K, Kanneganti S, Khajanchee Y, et al. The evolving role of staging laparoscopy in the treatment of colorectal hepatic metastasis. Arch Surg 2005;140:727–34.

[14] Milsom JW, Jerby BL, Kessler H, et al. Prospective, blinded comparison of laparoscopic ultrasonography vs. contrast-enhanced computerized tomography for liver assessment in patients undergoing colorectal carcinoma surgery. Dis Colon Rectum 2000;43:44–9.

[15] Machi J, Tateishi T, Oishi AJ, et al. Laparoscopic ultrasonography versus operative cholangiography during laparoscopic cholecystectomy: review of the literature and a comparison with open intraoperative ultrasonography. J Am Coll Surg 1999;188:360–7.

[16] Rothlin MA, Schlumpf R, Largiader F. Laparoscopic sonography. Arch Surg 1994;129:694–700.

[17] Azuma T, Yoshikawa T, Ariada T, et al. Intraoperative evaluation of the depth of invasion of gallbladder cancer. Am J Surg 1999;178:381–4.

[18] Taylor AM, Roberts SA, Manson JM. Experience with laparoscopic ultrasonography for defining tumour resectability in carcinoma of the pancreatic head and periampullary region. Br J Surg 2001;88:1077–83.

[19] Lo CY, Lo CM, Fan ST. Role of laparoscopic ultrasonography in intraoperative localization of pancreatic insulinoma. Surg Endosc 2000;14:1131–5.

[20] Ishihara M, Kanbe M, Okamoto T, et al. Laparoscopic ultrasonography for resection of insulinomas. Surgery 2001;130:1086–91.

[21] Schachter PP, Avni Y, Gvirz G, et al. The impact of laparoscopy and laparoscopic ultrasound on the management of pancreatic cystic lesions. Arch Surg 2000;135:260–4.

[22] Schachter PP, Shimonov M, Czerniak A. The role of laparoscopy and laparoscopic ultrasound in the diagnosis of cystic lesions of the pancreas. Gastrointest Endosc Clin North Am 2002;12:759–67.

[23] Brunt LM, Bennett HF, Teefey SA, et al. Laparoscopic ultrasound imaging of adrenal tumors during laparoscopic adrenalectomy. Am J Surg 1999;178:490–5.

[24] Helin HL, Kirkinen P. Laparoscopic ultrasonography during conservative ovarian surgery. Surg Endosc 2000;14:161–3.

[25] Noyan V, Tiras MB, Oktem M, et al. Laparoscopic ultrasonography in the management of ovarian cysts. Gynecol Obstet Invest 2005;60:63–6.

[26] Helin-Martikainen HL, Kirkinen P. Ultrasonography of the ureter during laparoscopic gynecological surgery. Ultrasound Obstet Gynecol 1997;9:414–8.

RADIOLOGIC
CLINICS
OF NORTH AMERICA

Radiol Clin N Am 44 (2006) 937–943

Index

Note: Page numbers of article titles are in **boldface** type.

doi:10.1016/S0033-8389(06)00123-0

United States Postal Service
Statement of Ownership, Management, and Circulation

1. Publication Title	2. Publication Number	3. Filing Date
Radiologic Clinics of North America	5 9 6 - 5 1 0	9/15/06

4. Issue Frequency	5. Number of Issues Published Annually	6. Annual Subscription Price
Jan, Mar, May, Jul, Sep, Nov	6	$235.00

7. Complete Mailing Address of Known Office of Publication (Not printer) (Street, city, county, state, and ZIP+4)

Elsevier Inc.
360 Park Avenue South
New York, NY 10010-1710

Contact Person
Sarah Carmichael
Telephone
(215) 239-3681

8. Complete Mailing Address of Headquarters or General Business Office of Publisher (Not printer)

Elsevier Inc., 360 Park Avenue South, New York, NY 10010-1710

9. Full Names and Complete Mailing Addresses of Publisher, Editor, and Managing Editor (Do not leave blank)

Publisher (Name and complete mailing address)

John Schrefer, Elsevier Inc., 1600 John F. Kennedy Blvd., Suite 1800, Philadelphia, PA 19103-2899

Editor (Name and complete mailing address)

Barton Dudlick, Elsevier Inc., 1600 John F. Kennedy Blvd., Suite 1800, Philadelphia, PA 19103-2899

Managing Editor (Name and complete mailing address)

Catherine Bewick, Elsevier Inc., 1600 John F. Kennedy Blvd., Suite 1800, Philadelphia, PA 19103-2899

10. Owner (Do not leave blank. If the publication is owned by a corporation, give the name and address of the corporation immediately followed by the names and addresses of all stockholders owning or holding 1 percent or more of the total amount of stock. If not owned by a corporation, give the names and addresses of the individual owners. If owned by a partnership or other unincorporated firm, give its name and address as well as those of each individual owner. If the publication is published by a nonprofit organization, give its name and address.)

Full Name	Complete Mailing Address
Wholly owned subsidiary of	4520 East-West Highway
Reed/Elsevier Inc., US Holdings	Bethesda, MD 20814

11. Known Bondholders, Mortgagees, and Other Security Holders Owning or Holding 1 Percent or More of Total Amount of Bonds, Mortgages, or Other Securities. If none, check box ▶ None

Full Name	Complete Mailing Address
N/A	

12. Tax Status (For completion by nonprofit organizations authorized to mail at nonprofit rates) (Check one)
The purpose, function, and nonprofit status of this organization and the exempt status for federal income tax purposes:
☐ Has Not Changed During Preceding 12 Months
☐ Has Changed During Preceding 12 Months (Publisher must submit explanation of change with this statement)

(See Instructions on Reverse)

PS Form 3526, October 1999

---

13. Publication Title		14. Issue Date for Circulation Data Below
Radiologic Clinics of North America		July, 2006

15.		Extent and Nature of Circulation	Average No. Copies Each Issue During Preceding 12 Months	No. Copies of Single Issue Published Nearest to Filing Date
a.		Total Number of Copies (Net press run)	7,750	7,700
b. Paid and/or Requested Circulation	(1)	Paid/Requested Outside-County Mail Subscriptions Stated on Form 3541. (Include advertiser's proof and exchange copies)	4,208	4,076
	(2)	Paid In-County Subscriptions Stated on Form 3541 (Include advertiser's proof and exchange copies)		
	(3)	Sales Through Dealers and Carriers, Street Vendors, Counter Sales, and Other Non-USPS Paid Distribution	2,132	2,287
	(4)	Other Classes Mailed Through the USPS		
c.		Total Paid and/or Requested Circulation [Sum of 15b. (1), (2), (3), and (4)] ▶	6,340	6,363
d. Free Distribution by Mail (Samples, compliment-ary, and other free)	(1)	Outside-County as Stated on Form 3541	171	206
	(2)	In-County as Stated on Form 3541		
	(3)	Other Classes Mailed Through the USPS		
e.		Free Distribution Outside the Mail (Carriers or other means)		
f.		Total Free Distribution (Sum of 15c. and 15e.) ▶	171	206
g.		Total Distribution (Sum of 15c. and 15f.) ▶	6,511	6,569
h.		Copies not Distributed	1,239	1,131
i.		Total (Sum of 15g. and h.) ▶	7,750	7,700
j.		Percent Paid and/or Requested Circulation (15c. divided by 15g. times 100)	97.37%	96.86%

16. Publication of Statement of Ownership
☑ Publication required. Will be printed in the **November 2006** issue of this publication. ☐ Publication not required

17. Signature and Title of Editor, Publisher, Business Manager, or Owner   Date

John Famucci - Executive Director of Subscription Services   9/15/06

I certify that all information furnished on this form is true and complete. I understand that anyone who furnishes false or misleading information on this form or who omits material or information requested on the form may be subject to criminal sanctions (including fines and imprisonment) and/or civil sanctions (including civil penalties).

Instructions to Publishers

1. Complete and file one copy of this form with your postmaster annually on or before October 1. Keep a copy of the completed form for your records.
2. In cases where the stockholder or security holder is a trustee, include in items 10 and 11 the name of the person or corporation for whom the trustee is acting. Also include the names and addresses of individuals who are stockholders who own or hold 1 percent or more of the total amount of bonds, mortgages, or other securities of the publishing corporation. In item 11, if none, check the box. Use blank sheets if more space is required.
3. Be sure to furnish all circulation information called for in item 15. Free circulation must be shown in items 15d, e, and f.
4. Item 15h, Copies not Distributed, must include (1) newsstand copies originally stated on Form 3541, and returned to the publisher, (2) estimated returns from news agents, and (3), copies for office use, leftovers, spoiled, and all other copies not distributed.
5. If the publication had Periodicals authorization as a general or requester publication, this Statement of Ownership, Management, and Circulation must be published; it must be printed in any issue in October or, if the publication is not published during October, the first issue printed after October.
6. In item 16, indicate the date of the issue in which this Statement of Ownership will be published.
7. Item 17 must be signed.
Failure to file or publish a statement of ownership may lead to suspension of Periodicals authorization.

PS Form 3526, October 1999 (Reverse)

Moving?

Make sure your subscription moves with you!

To notify us of your new address, find your **Clinics Account Number** (located on your mailing label above your name), and contact customer service at:

E-mail: elspcs@elsevier.com

800-654-2452 (subscribers in the U.S. & Canada)
407-345-4000 (subscribers outside of the U.S. & Canada)

Fax number: 407-363-9661

Elsevier Periodicals Customer Service
6277 Sea Harbor Drive
Orlando, FL 32887-4800

*To ensure uninterrupted delivery of your subscription, please notify us at least 4 weeks in advance of move.